W9-AKT-043

Parenting Children With ADHD

SECOND EDITION

Parenting Children With ADHD

10 Lessons That Medicine Cannot Teach

Vincent J. Monastra, PhD

American Psychological Association • Washington, DC

Copyright © 2014 by the American Psychological Association. All rights reserved. Except as permitted under the United States Copyright Act of 1976, no part of this publication may be reproduced or distributed in any form or by any means, including, but not limited to, the process of scanning and digitization, or stored in a database or retrieval system, without the prior written permission of the publisher.

Published by
APA LifeTools
750 First Street, NE
Washington, DC 20002
www.apa.org

To order
APA Order Department
P.O. Box 92984
Washington, DC 20090-2984
Tel: (800) 374-2721;
Direct: (202) 336-5510
Fax: (202) 336-5502;
TDD/TTY: (202) 336-6123
Online: www.apa.org/pubs/books
E-mail: order@apa.org

First Printing, February 2014
Second Printing, August 2017

In the U.K., Europe, Africa, and the Middle East, copies may be ordered from
American Psychological Association
3 Henrietta Street
Covent Garden, London
WC2E 8LU England

Typeset in Sabon by Circle Graphics, Inc., Columbia, MD

Printer: Bookmasters, Ashland, OH
Cover Designer: Naylor Design, Washington, DC

The opinions and statements published are the responsibility of the authors, and such opinions and statements do not necessarily represent the policies of the American Psychological Association.

Library of Congress Cataloging-in-Publication Data
Monastra, Vincent J., author.
  Parenting children with ADHD : 10 lessons that medicine cannot teach /
Vincent J. Monastra, PhD. — Second edition.
    pages cm
  Includes bibliographical references and index.
  ISBN-13: 978-1-4338-1571-3
  ISBN-10: 1-4338-1571-0
  1. Attention-deficit hyperactivity disorder—Treatment 2. Problem children—
Behavior modification. 3. Parenting. I. Title.

  RJ506.H9M65 2014
  618.92'8589—dc23
                                    2013045453

British Library Cataloguing-in-Publication Data
A CIP record is available from the British Library.

Printed in the United States of America
Second Edition

10 9 8 7 6 5 4 3 2

http://dx.doi.org/10.1037/14374-000

To God, from whom all wisdom comes.

CONTENTS

PREFACE TO THE SECOND EDITION

Ten years ago, I was sitting in front of this same computer, writing the first edition of *Parenting Children With ADHD: Ten Lessons That Medicine Cannot Teach*. When I stopped and looked back on all that has happened in my life since that time, I was amazed. So many changes in a decade. I guess that shouldn't have been a surprise to me, but it was. After all, in 10 years, a little kindergarten student goes from learning to ride a bike to learning to drive a car. In my case, my two big kids grew up, went off to college and became grownups. My two little kids came into my life, and my wife and I are back in the business of participating in PTA meetings, helping coach little-kid baseball teams, going to Vacation Bible School, and teaching our children about what matters most in life.

You too have gone through quite a change in the past 10 years. Maybe you have become a parent for the first time. Perhaps you have realized that you are the parent of a child with attention-deficit/hyperactivity disorder (ADHD). Or maybe you have spent a decade searching for a way to bring out the best in your child who has ADHD and felt like you were going nowhere. My hope is that what you learn from the second edition of my parenting book will guide you in raising a joyful, confident child who realizes that no one is perfect, that we all have talents, and that all of us can play an important role in making the world a much better and more loving place to live.

This edition has been updated to inform you about new developments in diagnosing ADHD, as well as new medications and psychological treatments for improving attention and helping your child be less impulsive and restless at home, school, and on the ball field. There have also been new initiatives in the field of education, the most important one being the emphasis on changing school environments from one in which bullying reigns to one in which respect for the dignity of all students is the new standard. This book will highlight those changes and guide you in ways to help your school district create a safe atmosphere for your child.

Finally, this book includes guidance for teaching life values. The previous edition provided a foundation for teaching new life skills. This edition expands on those lessons and offers a framework for teaching values like generosity, kindness, and compassion. As an attention disorders specialist, I thought it was important not only to help children improve their attention but also to encourage parents to reflect and teach what is actually most important. My hope is that you will.

Parenting
Children
With
ADHD

INTRODUCTION

In my early years as a psychologist, I found that most of the children I treated responded well to a combination of parental love and thoughtful administration of "consequences" for their actions. However, there were a small but significant number of kids who did not. These children would come into my office, week after week. Their parents would tell me about their efforts to get these children to listen, follow rules, remember chores, complete homework, clean their rooms, get along with their brothers and sisters, control their emotions, and develop friendships. Every session would seem the same. Although a child might have been able to improve in some small way, the session invariably turned into a review of his or her greatest "failures" for the week.

Even more torturous were the ensuing discussions in which the child would be asked to provide some explanation for her or his actions. If you have ever tried to have a discussion with a child who has attention-deficit/hyperactivity disorder (ADHD), you know what I am talking about. Sometimes kids with ADHD will go on and on and on, without ever getting to the point. Sometimes they will be so distracted that you need to repeatedly remind them of the question. Then, just when you're sure they have heard you, you'll get a brief answer like "I don't know" or a shrug. Other times they will "explode" and storm out of the room before you can get two words out. Even more amazing is the frequency of lying that occurs during discussions. I've witnessed conversations such as one in which a child denied he had broken a family rule and eaten chocolate before dinner, even though his hands and face were smeared with that tasty treat.

My watershed moment came during a 1-week period, approximately 25 years ago. It was the beginning of the summer. I was asked to evaluate two teenage boys. One boy's parents had begun the school year by offering their son the extraordinarily expensive "reward" of a new car based on his academic performance. The other boy's parents used a typical strategy of grounding their son from all social activities, television, and use of electronic games and computers until his grades improved. Which strategy do you think worked? The big bribe? The severe punishment? As it turned out, neither was effective.

Let's take a look at the parents who used the expensive reward. They told their son that if he could complete all his homework, attend all his classes, avoid disciplinary referrals to the principal, and merely pass each course for one marking period, they would buy him a new car. He failed to earn the car. After a year of prompting, prodding, encouraging, threatening, yelling, and crying, his parents brought him to me for treatment. Their poignant statement to me was, "Something must be seriously wrong with our son."

The other boy's parents took a different approach. In an effort to motivate their son to improve his grades, they restricted his activities. In essence, they told their son that he was "totally grounded": no calls, no contact with his friends after school or on the weekend, no involvement in school activities, no television, and no computer or video games. He was to spend his time completing his school assignments, studying, and resting for the next school day. Their deal was simple: Pass all courses for one marking period, and you are free. He never did. This teen was grounded for an entire year before he came to my office. I thought the family was kidding. One look at this teen's face told me the sad truth. This was no joke.

Think about the realities of these two stories for a minute. Put yourself in these teens' place. Let's say that your mom and dad offered to buy you a new car if you would go to school, stay out of trouble, complete and turn in your homework, and just pass your courses. I don't know about you, but I'd be talking with my folks about make, model, and color scheme for much of the first marking period and would be driving my new car by Thanksgiving. Turn it around. Let's say my folks "totally grounded me." Once I got over being furious, I would be determined to stay out of trouble, get my work done, and pass those stupid classes. There is no doubt in my mind that I could have done it. Same is true for you—if you don't have ADHD.

However, if you have ADHD, you, like my two teenage patients, would be bumming rides from friends or trying to sneak in a little television time. You'd continue to fail in school, prompting your parents and teachers to comment that you are unmotivated, have a poor attitude, and "could do better if you tried harder." At home, you would become increasingly distant from your parents, cutting yourself off from the most essential sources of love and self-confidence. As I have seen far too many times, the results in those situations are saddening, and sometimes tragic.

This book represents a compilation of the lessons I learned over the past three decades about ways to help children with ADHD succeed. It is an effort to synthesize the available medical, nutritional, educational, and psychological research into a format that can be used as a guidebook for parents or health care professionals conducting parenting class. It also provides a glimpse into how comprehensive clinical care can be provided in an outpatient setting, such as my clinic. A more detailed, scientific presentation of the research referenced in this book can be found in my 2008 book, *Unlocking the Potential of Patients With ADHD: A Model for Clinical Practice,* and in other references provided in the Supplemental Resources section of the book.

The second edition of *Parenting Children With ADHD: 10 Lessons That Medicine Cannot Teach* follows the structure of the Monastra ADHD Parenting Program (MAPP) provided at my clinic, with an emphasis placed on teaching parenting strategies, rather than providing a detailed presentation of the vast scientific literature in this field. The first 10 lessons in this book contain the material presented during parenting classes taught at my clinic. As a reader who hasn't had the benefit of participating in the live classes at my clinic, you also get two bonus lessons that discuss common problems experienced by parents as they work their way through the early stages of treatment with their children at my clinic.

As a clinical psychologist, directing the clinical research activities of my outpatient Attention Disorders Clinic, I have learned much by collaborating with psychiatrists, pediatricians, family practitioners, educators, counselors, and developmental specialists in the care of the approximately 15,000 patients seen at my clinic. My role has been to personally interview and review the medical and educational records of each of these children, provide psychological and electroencephalogram (EEG) evaluations, and then rely on the expertise of their physicians to determine the medical causes of the child's attention and behavioral control problems. Once that was done, the members of my clinical team and I have provided a wide range of clinical services, including parent counseling, EEG biofeedback, and social skills training for my patients. I also have helped physicians monitor a child's response to medication by providing quantitative EEG evaluations, neuropsychological testing, and collecting behavioral observations from parents and teachers when medications have been prescribed.

As you attempt to bring out the best in your child, you'll need the help of people who've been successful in treating children and teens with ADHD. Although you might not have a comprehensive center like my Attention Disorders Clinic in your city or town, chances are there are experienced therapists, educational consultants, psychologists, and physicians in your region who can be quite helpful. Your child's physician, a regional medical center, or the departments of psychology, psychiatry, social work, education, occupational, physical, and speech therapy at a college or university in your region are good resources to use as you put together your child's treatment team. Parent support groups such as Children and Adults with ADHD can also point you in the right direction.

As I developed our clinic's parenting program, I was struck by the complexity of the available materials and by how difficult it was to use this information in an organized manner. In a similar fashion, I was aware that a substantial number of my ADHD patients are parented by adults who also have ADHD. As a result, I have written this book as a series of sequential lessons to be taken one at a time. Because I realize that life at home can't come to a standstill until you read the next lesson, I have attempted to incorporate certain "lifelines" that you can use as you progress through this book.

I begin by sharing information about the causes of ADHD. I hope that as you learn about the biological factors that can cause problems of inattention, impulsivity, and hyperactivity in a child, you will be able to let go of any sense of guilt you may have regarding your role in causing your child's problems. As you come to understand the causes of ADHD, you will learn why the strategies other parents use to raise their children have failed with your child. ADHD is not a condition that will magically respond to any specific type of parental correction, nor will it be cured by any of the present forms of medical or psychological treatment.

ADHD is a condition that profoundly affects one's ability to succeed at home, school, and work and in social relationships. However, kids with ADHD can develop improved attention, behavioral control, and social skills. Although teachers, physicians, psychologists, and other health care providers can assist in your efforts to help your child succeed, in the end, you will realize that you are your child's best advocate and primary teacher in this process.

Initially, you and your child's physician will need to make sure that other kinds of medical problems are not interfering with your child's ability to listen, learn, and control his or her moods and actions. To help you understand the kinds of medical issues involved, I review other medical disorders that can cause impairment of attention, mood, and behavioral control. In addition, as part of your consultation with a physician, you will probably be asked to consider the range of medical interventions that can reduce the core symptoms of ADHD. Because medication issues are routinely discussed in the treatment of children with ADHD, I review the primary and secondary types of medical treatments to help you understand how these medications affect the underlying causes of ADHD. I will also let you know how doctors are beginning to use quantitative EEGs to better match children with type of medication to reduce the risk for side effects.

In addition to medical treatments, this book emphasizes the importance of other interventions that are needed to help your child. I review information regarding dietary factors and encourage you to examine the adequacy of your child's diet because certain foods are essential for mental functioning. I present a summary of educational laws and provide information to help you work collaboratively with your child's school district. I focus on helping you teach life skills and values that will help your child succeed on the playground, in the school, in the workplace, and, one day, as a spouse and parent. I also describe effective psychological treatments for promoting your child's attention, memory, problem-solving ability, and social development. Finally, because "parents are people too," I explore ways to create time and space for you to enjoy some pleasurable moments with your child, friends, and loved ones. To help you apply the lessons contained in this book, I have included various worksheets, charts, and checklists. Feel free to photocopy these forms for your personal use only. You can also download forms from the book's companion website: http://pubs.apa.org/books/supp/monastra.

One last thought before you begin. In my work with parents, I have noted three traits that breed success. First, the parents who report the most progress in their children take it one lesson at a time and do their homework. These parents accept the reality that they will not be able to make headway on all of their children's problems at once. They focus on the goals of a particular lesson, and they follow through. Second, my most successful parents remember that lessons learned in one class need to be continued as the course progresses. They usually have a game plan that they review weekly and continue to do so on an ongoing basis. Third, parents whose kids succeed are persistent. If things are not working out the way they hoped, they ask questions, seek clarification, and revise their approach.

You may be wondering, "What's the payoff?" I had that question too. So I studied the outcomes of children treated at my clinic and looked closely at parenting style. A scientific paper that describes this study in detail was published in the journal *Applied Psychophysiology and Biofeedback* (see Supplemental Readings for details). First, I made sure that all the children in the study had been thoroughly evaluated for ADHD (and other medical problems) and were being treated with medication for their ADHD. I then took the time to work with schools to develop support programs for each of these children. During this process, parents began our parenting program. At the end of a year, their children's progress was evaluated. The results indicated that parents who systematically used the lessons taught in this book had children who showed significantly fewer symptoms of ADHD at home. My hope is that you will have similar success with your child.

As you read this book, you may find yourself wanting more detailed information about a particular topic. To help you in your search, I have included a listing of selected books and scientific papers. These supplemental readings are listed by lesson and can be found at the end of the book. With that said, let's get started.

EVERYBODY DOESN'T HAVE A LITTLE BIT OF ADHD

As a typical American, prone to surfing through the channels on my television, I have often witnessed the following scene. Two chairs. Coffee table. Plastic flowers. Books in the background. One reporter. One expert in the studio (the advocate expert). One expert (with an opposing viewpoint) is available via satellite for comment. The topic: attention-deficit/hyperactivity disorder (ADHD).

Invariably, the in-studio expert is asked to define ADHD. This doctor provides some variation of the following statement:

> ADHD is a psychiatric disorder characterized by symptoms of inattention, with or without evidence of hyperactivity. Some of these symptoms were noticed by age 12. The condition does not usually disappear with age; it is likely to cause impairment throughout a person's life. Patients diagnosed with ADHD are inattentive, seem to act without thinking, fail to listen to instructions, and have difficulty concentrating at school and completing their schoolwork. They are at risk out of dropping out of school, using illegal drugs, and eventually having difficulty succeeding at work and in their marriages.

The advocate expert typically proceeds to present the case that ADHD is a "real" medical condition that is inherited, and he or she makes reference to some kind of biochemical "imbalance" that causes the disorder.

Next, the opposing side is heard. This expert offers comments that suggest "everyone has a bit of ADHD." The expert contends that ADHD is a condition that has been dreamed up by pharmaceutical companies and a group of doctors who have conspired to make billions of dollars by selling drugs to kids. Typically, this expert makes some reference to the dangers of promoting addiction in children and excusing them from accepting responsibility for their actions. Sometimes an anthropological spin is presented, which suggests that kids with ADHD are like hunters living in a society that no longer needs that type of service. The conclusion of the interview consists of a listing of ADHD symptoms with a recommendation that if your child shows these symptoms, you should consult with his or her physician.

At first glance, that conclusion may sound OK. However, it skirts the real issue. Is ADHD really a medical condition that requires treatment? Or is it just a term used by people to avoid responsibility or to drug kids and make tons of money? To answer these questions, the National Institutes of Health (NIH) organized a meeting in 1998, the NIH Consensus Conference on the Diagnosis and Treatment of ADHD. (The complete Consensus Statement is available on the NIH website; see Supplemental Resources). During this 3-day meeting, hundreds of ADHD specialists, including myself, met in Bethesda, Maryland, to review the scientific evidence regarding the causes and treatments for ADHD. Because ADHD is one of the most extensively researched disorders in our society, the NIH was able to examine the results of more than a thousand scientific studies. On the basis of this review, the NIH concluded that ADHD was indeed a health impairment that (when untreated) increased a person's risk for failure at school, involvement in substance abuse and criminal activities, and the development of a variety of problems at work and in social relationships.

ADHD is a condition that is diagnosed on the basis of the presence of a degree of inattention or hyperactivity and impulsivity that is so great it interferes with a person's ability to succeed at home, school, work, or in relationships with others. Physicians, psychologists, and other qualified health care professionals diagnose ADHD according to the presence of symptoms that listed in the fifth edition of the *Diagnostic and Statistical Manual of Mental Disorders* (*DSM–5;* American Psychiatric Association, 2013). For a person to be diagnosed with ADHD, he or she must meet five separate standards (called *criteria*). These criteria have to do with the number of symptoms, the age at which these symptoms first caused difficulties, the situations in which these symptoms are shown, and the presence of impairment of functioning at school, at work, or in social relationships. In addition, it must be shown that these symptoms are not caused by another mental or physical disorder.[1]

THE FIVE CRITERIA NEEDED TO DIAGNOSE ADHD

The first criterion for a diagnosis of ADHD has to do with the number of symptoms of inattention, hyperactivity, or impulsivity shown by a person. Strange as it may sound, not all patients with ADHD will show symptoms of inattention. Similarly, not all patients with ADHD will be hyperactive, which is confusing. *To be diagnosed with ADHD, a child must show at least six symptoms of inattention, impulsivity, or hyperactivity. Children 17 and older (and adults) must show at least five symptoms of inattention, impulsivity, or hyperactivity. These symptoms must have been observed for at least 6 months.* If the child only shows a sufficient number of symptoms of inattention, they meet one of the criteria for the diagnosis of ADHD, *Predominately Inattentive Presentation.*

---

[1]From the *Diagnostic and Statistical Manual of Mental Disorders, Fifth Edition,* 2013. Copyright 2013 by the American Psychiatric Association. Reprinted with permission.

If they only show a sufficient number of symptoms of hyperactivity-impulsivity, they meet one of the criteria for the diagnosis of ADHD, *Predominately Hyperactive-Impulsive Presentation*. If they show enough symptoms of both inattention and hyperactivity-impulsivity, they meet the first criteria to be diagnosed with ADHD, *Combined Presentation*.

This definition of the subtypes of ADHD can be pretty confusing, so many people use the term *ADD* (attention-deficit disorder) when the patient only has problems with attention and the term *ADHD* when hyperactivity is also a problem. My guess is that will continue to occur in conversations and media discussions about ADHD. However, the current manual used by physicians, psychologists, and other mental health professionals (*DSM–5*) lists ADHD, Predominately Inattentive Presentation; ADHD, Predominately Hyperactive-Impulsive Presentation; and ADHD, Combined Presentation as the primary kinds of ADHD. Throughout this book, whenever the term *ADHD* is used, it refers to children and teens who meet the criteria for any of the three types of ADHD.

Following is the *DSM–5* definition of the symptoms of ADHD.

Inattention

Nine types of inattentive behaviors are listed in the *DSM–5*. The patient must show the behavior "often" for it to be considered cause for concern. The behaviors are described in the following way:

a. fails to give close attention to details or makes careless mistakes in schoolwork, work, or other activities (e.g., overlooks or misses details, work is inaccurate);

b. has difficulty sustaining attention in tasks or play activities (e.g., has difficulty remaining focused during lectures, conversations, or lengthy reading);

c. does not seem to listen when spoken to directly (e.g., mind seems elsewhere, even in the absence of any obvious distraction);

d. does not follow through on instructions and fails to finish schoolwork, chores, or duties in the workplace (e.g., starts tasks but quickly loses focus and is easily sidetracked);
e. has difficulty organizing tasks and activities (e.g., difficulty managing sequential tasks; difficulty keeping materials and belongings in order; messy, disorganized work; has poor time management; fails to meet deadlines);
f. avoids, dislikes, or is reluctant to engage in tasks that require sustained mental effort (e.g., schoolwork or homework; for older adolescents and adults, preparing reports, completing forms, reviewing lengthy papers);
g. loses things necessary for tasks or activities (e.g., school materials, pencils, books, tools, wallets, keys, paperwork, eyeglasses, mobile telephones);
h. is easily distracted by extraneous stimuli (for older adolescents and adults, may include unrelated thoughts); and
i. is forgetful in daily activities (e.g., doing chores, running errands; for older adolescents and adults, returning calls, paying bills, keeping appointments).

Hyperactivity-Impulsivity

There are nine types of hyperactive-impulsive behaviors listed in the *DSM–5* used by physicians, psychologists, and other licensed mental health providers. As with inattentive behaviors, a child must show at least six of these nine symptoms "often" to meet the first criterion for a diagnosis of ADHD. Again, children ages 17 and older only need to show at least five "hyperactive" or "impulsive" symptoms. The specific behaviors are described in the following way:

a. fidgets with or taps hands or feet or squirms in seat;
b. leaves seat in situations in which remaining seated is expected (e.g., leaves his or her place in the classroom, in the office or

other workplace, or in other situations that require remaining in place);

c. runs about or climbs in situations in which it is inappropriate (in adolescents or adults, may be limited to feeling restless);

d. unable to play or engage in leisure activities quietly;

e. is "on the go," acting as if "driven by a motor" (e.g., is unable to be or is uncomfortable being still for extended time, as in restaurants, meetings; may be experienced by others as being restless or difficult to keep up with);

f. talks excessively;

g. blurts out an answer before a question has been completed (e.g., completes people's sentences; cannot wait for turn in conversation);

h. has difficulty waiting his or her turn (e.g., while waiting in line); and

i. interrupts or intrudes on others (e.g., butts into conversations, games, or activities; may start using other people's things without asking or receiving permission; for adolescents, may intrude into or take over what others are doing).

So to determine whether your child has ADHD, he or she needs to have at least six symptoms of inattention, six of hyperactivity-impulsivity, or a combination of six of each type of symptom (12 total). If this seems true about your child, then she or he meets part of the first criterion for this diagnosis.

An equally important part of this first criterion is that the symptoms of inattention, impulsivity, or hyperactivity are occurring more frequently than would be expected for the child's age. Because of the need to compare a child's behavior with that of other children, doctors often ask parents, teachers, and others who are familiar with a child to complete "behavioral rating" questionnaires. These forms ask a person to provide information about the kinds of ADHD symptoms that they observe and the frequency with which these symptoms occur. If the ratings provided by parents or others indicate that the frequency of a child's inattentive, hyperactive, or impulsive behaviors is greater than 93% of their peers, then the test results are considered to be supportive of a diagnosis of ADHD. Doctors typically require that a child demonstrate a symptom frequency greater than 93% of peers to consider diagnosing a patient with any type of illness or condition. Although the results of these rating forms alone are not sufficient to determine a diagnosis of ADHD, they do provide a useful way to compare a child's behavior with that of other children of the same age.

The second criterion for the diagnosis of ADHD concerns the child's age when symptoms first started to become apparent. *For a doctor to diagnose ADHD, several ADHD symptoms had to be present before 12 years of age.* This does not mean that the child had to be diagnosed with ADHD before age 12. It just means that some symptoms of inattention, impulsivity, or hyperactivity had to be observed by that age.

The requirement that the child needs to show several symptoms of ADHD by the age of 12 makes a lot more sense than the "rule" listed in previous diagnostic manuals. Before *DSM–5*, the child needed to show symptoms by age 7. However, in many children, serious concerns about attention wouldn't occur until the second or third grade, when the child was struggling to complete homework. Even then, many parents would just naturally start to take over and function as their child's brain for years, repeatedly reminding the child about responsibilities, helping the child stay organized, endlessly explaining family rules, and working for hours on end to help their child keep on top of homework. Because the parents did so, their son or daughter continued to earn good grades throughout primary school. Thus, it often wasn't until the child was in middle school and unable to do homework or take notes during lectures or was disruptive in class that significant problems were apparent to parents and teachers.

Over the years, clinical researchers have learned that although some children with ADHD are diagnosed by age 7, others are identified at later ages. In reviewing my clinical records, I found several primary periods when children are referred for an evaluation for ADHD. The first occurs between 3 and 5 years of age. These children are impulsive and hyperactive. Their parents or guardians are typically terrified about potential injuries that could occur because of their child's behavior, exhausted by the demands of protecting their child, and at a loss to explain why the kinds of discipline that work for everybody else's kids don't work for them.

The second period occurs toward the end of the primary grades (about third grade). At this age, I begin to receive referrals to evaluate children who struggle to maintain attention and concentration and who are having difficulties completing school assignments. In addition, hyperactive children who were considered simply immature at 5 or 6 years of age begin to be referred for evaluation because their behavior is severely disruptive in the classroom.

The third period occurs during middle school years. Both inattentive and hyperactive-impulsive children who are failing to succeed in school despite repeated teacher conferences and parental discipline are referred during this time. These children are typically considered unmotivated or emotionally disturbed. Children who are inattentive are suspected of being depressed because they have few friends, engage in little spontaneous conversation, and show little response to rewards or punishments. Children whose behavior is hyperactive-impulsive are suspected of having bipolar disorder, a conduct disorder, or an oppositional-defiant disorder because they lie, argue with parents, defy parental and school rules, and display frequent outbursts of temper.

The fourth period occurs in high school, when a child has been repeatedly suspended from school and appears at risk for dropout.

These children are rarely referred by a school district but rather by parents who have seen a television program on ADHD or who have read a book, magazine article, or story about ADHD and have begun to realize that their child had many symptoms of the disorder but was never diagnosed.

These are the kids whose kindergarten teachers had described as exuberant, full of energy, and creative. They had teachers in the primary grades who recognized their intelligence but were concerned because the children had difficulty listening, following directions, concentrating, and completing assignments. By the middle school years, these same children were described as unmotivated. They are the children who "could do better if they tried harder." They are told that "they should be able to" take notes, read textbooks for essential details, study, and complete their assignments. If the children are tested for learning disabilities, their parents are told they do not qualify for help because they do not have learning disabilities in reading, mathematics, or writing (I examine this issue more fully in Lesson 5). These children often misbehave in class, are frequently truant, are disciplined for violating school policies, and are repeatedly punished by their parents.

The final period in which children are referred to me is after high school. Among these patients are young adults with incredibly committed parents who worked tirelessly to address their children's problems of inattention, disorganization, and failure to complete schoolwork. These young adults commonly report that their parents would devote 4 to 8 hours per day helping them study and complete homework. These patients often had tutors on a daily basis. However, when they began to attend college, their problems attending, taking notes, comprehending while reading, writing, and studying surfaced. These students, who were frequently on the honor roll in high school, are typically floundering to pass college-level courses, and their parents are at a loss to explain why.

The other group of patients referred after high school are young adults who have developed significant substance abuse or legal problems, yet their parents are convinced that they are not bad kids. These children have typically dropped out of college, have a pattern of being fired or quitting jobs, have little money, and display highly aggressive and abusive behavior toward their parents. Their parents are likely to have recently "discovered" ADHD and recognized a pattern of inattention, impulsivity, or hyperactivity that began in early childhood. These parents almost hope that their children have this disorder so they will finally have a diagnosis to explain their children's behaviors.

Because of research published in this area, health care professionals understand that there is no age limit for diagnosing ADHD. The diagnosis is not restricted to early childhood. It does not need to be made during grade school or even by the conclusion of high school. The condition can persist and interfere with a person's success throughout his or her life. *Consequently, regardless of your child's age, if some ADHD symptoms were causing problems at home or at school by age 12, the child meets the second criterion for a diagnosis of ADHD.*

The third criterion for a diagnosis of ADHD requires that *several symptoms are present in two or more settings (e.g., at home, school, or work; with friends or relatives; in other activities).* This does not mean that the results of behavioral rating scales must show that the frequency of symptoms is greater than 93% of peers at home and at school. It means that evidence of ADHD symptoms needs to be observed in more than one setting. So if you have to repeat your instructions to your son or daughter over and over again, if you have to remind your daughter a million times not to do something (but she keeps doing it), or if your child keeps losing his lunchbox, coat, sneakers, or toys, then he or she is showing symptoms of ADHD at home. Similarly, if your child seems unable to focus in class, forgets to write down assignments, completes but somehow forgets to turn in assignments, or is constantly interrupting class, then he or she is showing symptoms of ADHD at school. The child who demonstrates several symptoms of ADHD at home and at school would meet the third criterion for a diagnosis of ADHD.

The fourth criterion for a diagnosis of ADHD requires that *there is clear evidence that the symptoms interfere with, or reduce the quality of, social, academic, or occupational functioning.* An obvious question is, what is clear evidence? Here are a couple of examples. Certainly, the presence of failing grades in school qualifies if the child has at least average intelligence. In addition, depending on grade expectations, if a child is unable to record homework assignments, bring home necessary materials, take notes in class, read textbooks for detail and understanding, complete written assignments, prepare study guides, and study for tests because of attention problems, these can be considered a sign of functional impairment. So can a child's lack of friends, difficulties in resolving peer conflicts, or inability to engage in meaningful conversations. On a day-to-day level, if your child is experiencing anger (instead of praise and acceptance) because she or he is careless, fails to attend, does not listen, is disorganized, avoids homework, and so on, then these symptoms interfere with functioning at home. Similarly, if your child is being prevented from playing at recess; is being detained after school to complete school-work; is being scolded, belittled, or reprimanded; is being removed from class; or is receiving failing grades because of ADHD symptoms, then his or her symptoms are interfering with functioning at school. If these types of problems are occurring with your child, then your child meets the fourth criterion for a diagnosis of ADHD.

In my opinion, the fifth and final criterion for ADHD is often ignored or minimized by health care professionals. *It requires that the doctor diagnosing ADHD determines the symptoms of inattention, impulsivity, or hyperactivity are not caused by another mental or physical disorder.* We live in an era in which the need for laboratory tests is closely scrutinized, and there is a tendency to question the need for blood tests or other diagnostic procedures before determining a diagnosis of ADHD. I have real concerns when physicians fail to order or insurance companies fail to approve certain laboratory tests, and I strongly recommend that patients receive a thorough physical evaluation for all medical conditions that can be contributing to their attention problems. Here's why.

Did you know that symptoms of inattention are a characteristic of hypoglycemia? of anemia? of diabetes? of thyroid disorders? of sleep apnea? of allergies? of insufficiencies of vitamin D, vitamin B, zinc, calcium, and magnesium? Are you aware that school-age children and teens who get insufficient sleep and skip breakfast will have problems sustaining attention, concentrating in class, recalling information, and completing assignments simply because of dietary and sleep deficits? Are you aware that a child's difficulty completing reading or writing tasks could be caused by difficulties in visual tracking and convergence that are not easily detected in a routine eye examination of visual acuity? Maybe you are, but maybe you aren't. I was surprised to find that at least 10% to 20% of patients screened for ADHD at our clinic each year had one of these problems. If you aren't aware that problems of inattention, hyperactivity, and impulsivity can be caused by medical problems other than ADHD, I'd encourage you to take a look at my book *Unlocking the Potential of Patients With ADHD: A Model for Clinical Practice*, any standard medical text (e.g., *Cecil's Textbook of Medicine*), or search WebMD (or another reputable medical website). I think you'd be amazed at what you discover.

Your doctor is, or should be, aware that the conditions listed here (and other conditions as well) can and do cause symptoms of inattention, impulsivity, and hyperactivity. Although I have now participated in the evaluation and treatment of thousands of patients with significant problems in attention or behavioral control, I have rarely encountered a patient who had been screened for these conditions prior to seeing me. In fact, it is not uncommon for a physician to inform me that she or he did not screen for these conditions because there was no medical reason to do so. I respectfully disagree. Because patients suspected of ADHD have a significant problem attending and patients with each of the other medical problems I listed also have significant attention problems, I think there is sufficient cause to evaluate a patient for other medical problems. So does the *DSM–5*.

The guidelines established by the American Psychiatric Association require that a physician, psychologist, or other mental health provider make sure that another medical condition is not causing the ADHD-like symptoms. The *DSM–5* states that "visual and hearing impairments, metabolic abnormalities, sleep disorders, nutritional deficiencies, and epilepsy should be considered as possible influences on ADHD symptoms." Tests for these conditions are reliable, relatively inexpensive, and readily available; I advocate their use. During presentations to physicians, psychologists, and other mental health care providers, I ask how they would feel if they discovered that a patient they treated for ADHD actually had sleep apnea, dietary insufficiencies, hypoglycemia, a thyroid disorder, a vitamin D deficiency, a visual tracking or convergence disorder, or other medical condition? I have to ask parents and guardians the same question. Once you are assured that your child's symptoms are not attributable to another medical problem, you are ready for the next step.

HOMEWORK

Before reading the next lesson, take a little time to digest this information. In this lesson, I gave you a summary of the components required for a diagnosis of ADHD. If you suspect that your child meets these criteria but has not been evaluated for ADHD or the other medical conditions that can cause such symptoms, make arrangements to have such an evaluation completed. Similarly, if your child has been diagnosed with ADHD but has not been evaluated for other medical conditions that could cause these symptoms, I encourage you to obtain such a medical evaluation. To help you, your psychologist, or other mental health provider request a comprehensive medical evaluation, I have provided an example of the letter that I use at my clinic. Although it may represent a slight inconvenience for you and your child to go through this process, in the end, if your child happens to be among the children who have other medical causes for their ADHD symptoms, it may be the smartest move you ever made.

Request For Medical Evaluation

DATE: _____

PATIENT: _____   **BIRTHDATE:** ____

Dear Dr. _____,

This patient has recently been evaluated because of symptoms suggestive of ADHD. On the basis of a comprehensive review of the patient's medical, developmental, educational, and social histories, as well as the results of behavioral rating scales and neuropsychological testing of attention and executive functions, this patient has been diagnosed with ADHD, pending medical evaluation by your office. A copy of my evaluation report will be forwarded to you.

Because symptoms of inattention and impaired behavioral and emotional control can be caused by medical conditions other than ADHD, I have recommended that this patient be evaluated by you to rule out the following medical conditions that can cause inattention and loss of behavioral and emotional control:

- anemia
- sleep disorder (apnea; deficits)
- thyroid disorders
- hypoglycemia
- diabetes
- zinc deficiency
- magnesium deficiency
- calcium deficiency
- vitamin D deficiency
- vitamin B deficiency (B1, B3, B9, B12)
- illegal psychoactive substance use (teens, adults)
- Food allergies (e.g., corn, wheat, gluten, eggs, dairy, cocoa, nuts, food dyes)

To provide effective clinical care for this patient, I would appreciate your assistance in conducting whatever laboratory and clinical assessments you consider necessary to rule out these conditions before initiating treatment for ADHD.

Thank you for your assistance.

_____

Name of Referring Provider

© Vincent J. Monastra, PhD

LESSON 2

PARENTING DOESN'T CAUSE ADHD, GENES DO!

As I noted in Lesson 1, there has been much public debate about the causes of attention-deficit/hyperactivity disorder (ADHD). Some Americans believe that ADHD is a fictional condition, created by pharmaceutical companies and doctors to drum up business. Others consider it to be a condition caused by parents who spoil their children. Still others note the reactions of children to certain foods (e.g., wheat, corn), food dyes, or preservatives and argue that dietary habits are responsible for ADHD.

The scientific evidence available at this time indicates that none of these are true; however, like any type of opinion, there is a bit of truth underlying each position. Corporate greed can be a problem in any business endeavor. "Spoiling" does not help the development of any child, but there is no evidence that parenting style causes ADHD. Similarly, although certain children do display symptoms of inattention, impulsivity, or hyperactivity because of allergies (or other medical problems), ADHD is a distinct medical condition that by definition is not caused by other medical or psychiatric disorders.

As I mentioned in Lesson 1, ADHD is not diagnosed simply by the presence of inattention, impulsivity, or hyperactivity. Because various medical conditions can cause such symptoms, the diagnosis also requires medical evaluation to rule out the presence of other health problems with symptoms that mimic ADHD. For example, patients with diabetes can routinely experience difficulties in concentrating if they ignore dietary recommendations or fail to follow their physician's orders regarding the use of medication. However, doctors don't call their condition ADHD. Patients who have anemia can be forgetful, easily fatigued, unable to concentrate and attend to task, and can become disorganized and irritable. Again, doctors don't say that a person with anemia has ADHD. This is also the case for individuals with other medical conditions such as hypoglycemia, thyroid disorders, certain types of allergies, sleep disorders and deficiencies of vitamin D, calcium, zinc, and magnesium. Such symptoms can also be noted in children who have visual problems, hearing loss, and specific learning disabilities (e.g., reading, mathematics, written expression). Because multiple medical pathways can lead to symptoms of inattention, hyperactivity, or impulsivity, the mere presence of these symptoms does not mean that a person has ADHD.

The diagnosis of ADHD requires that doctors conduct thorough evaluations of patients to determine what is causing these symptoms. If a patient has at least six symptoms of inattention or hyperactivity-impulsivity (or both) and these symptoms have been present since at least age 12 years, have been observed in at least two settings (e.g., home, school, community), are causing significant functional problems in at least one of these settings, and are not due to any other medical condition, then a diagnosis of ADHD can be determined. However, knowing this does not help us really understand why 5% to 10% of American children have problems attending, concentrating, and controlling their actions despite the efforts of their parents and teachers.

SO WHAT IS ADHD?

ADHD is a psychiatric condition that has been primarily associated with a pattern of inactivity in the frontal lobes of the brain. The *Diagnostic and Statistical Manual of Mental Disorders (DSM–5)* notes that "as a group, compared with peers, children with ADHD display increased slow wave electroencephalograms, reduced total brain volume on magnetic resonance imaging, and possibly a delay in posterior to anterior cortical maturation." This basically means that the part of the person's body that is in charge of thinking, planning, concentrating, retrieving information, and staying on task is not as active as it needs to be for a person to succeed at school, work, and home. When children, teens, and adults with ADHD have been examined with a variety of brain-imaging techniques (e.g., positron emission tomography [PET] scans, single-photon emission computed tomography [SPECT] scans, functional magnetic resonance imaging [fMRI], or quantitative electroencephalography [QEEG]), a pattern of "underarousal" has been evident in the vast majority of these patients.

Beginning in the early 1990s, published scientific reports have revealed that patients with ADHD show a slowing in the rate that glucose (sugar) is used in the frontal lobes. We also have learned that a slowing of oxygen flow into the frontal lobes typically occurs in patients with ADHD. Finally, when the electrical "output" of brain cells is examined on quantitative QEEGs, this same pattern of slowing is noted in the electrical activity of brain cells in this region.

The electroencephalography research has been so compelling that in 2013, the U.S. Food and Drug Administration (FDA) determined that a QEEG–based test (neuropsychiatric EEG-based assessment aid, or NEBA), founded on the process developed and patented by Dr. Joel Lubar and myself, was approved for use in the diagnosis of ADHD. Although there is extensive research support for use of this test, some psychologists and psychiatrists who treat ADHD have expressed concerns about the cost of using this procedure. Before I comment on this, it should be noted that I do have a vested interest in the development and use of this process. However, parents also need to be aware that the cost of a QEEG evaluation is similar to the expense of a clinical interview, administration and interpretation of behavioral rating scales, and other psychological and neuropsychological tests used in clinical practice (ranging from $175 to $1,000, depending on the type of QEEG used). It is also important for parents to be aware that the FDA decided to approve this test because it improved the accuracy of the doctor's diagnosis. Improved accuracy translates to better treatment response and lower health care costs. As insurance companies become more aware of the FDA's decision, we hope they will provide coverage for this type of evaluation.

What Causes This Inactivity in the Brain?

The application of neuroimaging technology has greatly increased understanding of how underarousal of the brain may occur. Scientists have long known that brain cells communicate by releasing certain chemicals called *neurotransmitters*. For a message to be sent and received by other cells, a bit of neurotransmitter must be released, avoid being reabsorbed by a reuptake transport system (that attempts to bring released neurotransmitters back into the cell), travel across a space between cells called a *synapse*, and activate docking stations or *receptors* on the nearby brain cells. If sufficient activation of the nearby cell occurs, then that cell releases neurotransmitters, and the process of communication continues.

Take a few minutes to look at the illustration in Figure 2.1. You'll notice that the picture of the brain highlights the frontal lobe (particularly, the prefrontal cortex). This is the region of the brain

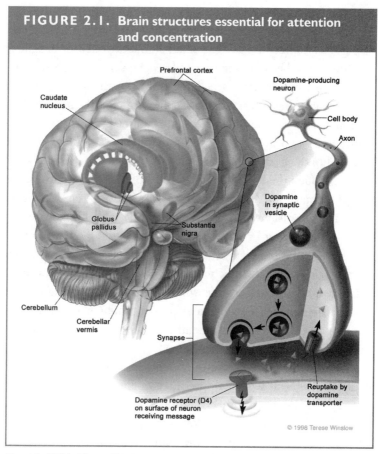

FIGURE 2.1. Brain structures essential for attention and concentration

Copyright 1998 by Therese Winslow. Reprinted with permission.

that is important for attention, concentration, and working memory. When it is activated, your child is able to block out distractions and create enough mental energy to concentrate on one task at a time. However, when this region is not sufficiently activated, your child will be unable to focus on your instructions, understand what he or she is reading, or think before acting.

The way that brain cells communicate is illustrated by the adjacent picture of a single transmitting cell and a nearby receiving cell. The transmitter cell is releasing small amounts of neurotransmitter into the space between the two cells (synapse). You can see particles of neurotransmitter attaching to the dopamine receptor and other particles being reabsorbed. The brain chemicals that attach to dopamine receptors cause the awakening of the brain. Those neurotransmitters that are reabsorbed by the dopamine transporter get returned to the transmitting cell for later use.

Although there are numerous types of neurotransmitters, the one of primary interest in studies of ADHD has been dopamine. Other neurotransmitters (e.g., norepinephrine, epinephrine) are also involved in helping us take notice of what's going on around us, keeping us still, and enabling us to focus on one thing, block out sources of distraction, and concentrate, understand, and remember what we are sensing. These neurotransmitters are found in regions of the brain that are involved in attention, thinking, and control of our moods and movements, primarily in the frontal lobes, the sensorimotor cortex, and the cerebellum.

Neurotransmitters like dopamine are manufactured in our bodies from foods with high protein content, such as meats, fish, poultry, eggs, dairy products, certain beans (e.g., soy), and nuts. This manufacturing process takes place primarily in the morning and early afternoon. Although the body is capable of storing a certain amount of dopamine, the truth is that if we fail to eat a breakfast that includes a sufficient amount of protein, we will have difficulty concentrating by mid-morning, whether we have ADHD or not. If the first time during the day that a person eats protein is at lunch, it is likely that he or she will feel quite sluggish and inattentive within an hour of lunchtime.

Because of the connection between dietary protein and attention, one of the aspects of treatment I emphasize is finding a way to get at least 15 to 20 grams of protein into a patient's breakfast and lunch. I review strategies for improving nutrition in Lesson 4. However, it is important to realize that consuming a sufficient amount of protein will not "cure" ADHD. What it will do is make it possible for a patient's brain cells to have an adequate supply of dopamine (and other neurotransmitters) to "communicate" with other brain cells.

We have learned that ADHD is not caused by an insufficient amount of dopamine. Instead, the problem appears to be related to what happens when a brain cell tries to release dopamine to "talk" to other brain cells. There is evidence that patients with ADHD have a reuptake system that reabsorbs about 70% more of the released dopamine than people who don't have ADHD. That means the brain cells of patients with ADHD are transmitting far less neurotransmitter to nearby cells than people who don't have ADHD. In addition, there is evidence that the brain cells that are receiving dopamine have approximately 16% fewer "docking" sites (receptors). The result is that nearby cells are not being activated as quickly. This underactivity is what is evident on QEEG scans, PET scans, SPECT scans, and fMRI. Current scientific evidence suggests that this neurological underactivity is what causes patients with ADHD to have difficulty sustaining attention, concentration, thinking, regulating their emotional responses, and controlling their behavior.

In a sense, the children who have inherited these characteristics have what I call the *smart brain* or the *energy-saver* brain. Instead of launching into full, sustained attention in low-excitement situations (e.g., picking up their stuff, remembering their chores, copying spelling words, reading boring books, learning uninteresting scientific or historical facts, and recording and completing their homework), the brains of children with ADHD seem to be monitoring their surroundings, attending to events that are important, interesting, life-threatening, or fun, ignoring those that aren't. If the situation is important, interesting, life-threatening, or fun, then regions of the brain that are involved in helping us pursue pleasure and avoid pain rev up the frontal lobes. Now their brain cells' ability to rapidly reabsorb dopamine turns into an advantage because they can more quickly fire, reload, and fire again. As a result, kids with ADHD can really pay attention and outperform most other people when they're doing something they like or in high-risk situations.

Do All Children With ADHD Show Underarousal of the Frontal Lobes?

No. Over the past 2 decades, a series of studies using QEEG procedures have revealed that approximately 10% to 20% of patients with ADHD do not show excessive cortical slowing over brain regions responsible for sustained attention and concentration. Interestingly, this research has also suggested that that this type of patient tends to respond poorly to stimulant medications. It is unclear whether patients in this neurological "subgroup" of ADHD (who demonstrate excessive activity over frontal regions) actually have ADHD or if they have another type of neurological disorder characterized by symptoms of inattention, impulsivity, and hyperactivity. When I talk to children and teens about their experience when they are inattentive, those who have underarousal of the frontal lobes describe it as more of a loss of awareness—kind of "blanking out." Those who have hyperarousal over the frontal lobes indicate that they are distracted by other thoughts when they are trying to concentrate on something.

How Did My Child Get This Condition?

Although children who experience prenatal exposure to alcohol, heroin, or cocaine; birth trauma; or lead poisoning are likely to have attention and other neurodevelopmental problems, I consider it inaccurate when such children are diagnosed with ADHD. Similarly, I think it is inaccurate to use the term ADHD if attention and behavioral problems are shown by patients with diabetes, hypoglycemia, thyroid disorders, anemia, allergies, sleep apnea, vitamin D deficiency, and other medical conditions. Only if the ADHD symptoms persisted after these medical conditions were adequately treated would I consider a diagnosis of ADHD to be appropriate.

The current understanding of ADHD is that it is an inherited condition. ADHD occurs in approximately 5% of the American population. However, that rate increases dramatically in families where there is at least one parent who also has this disorder. About 57% of adults with ADHD will have at least one child with this condition. If you have a child who has been diagnosed with ADHD, the chance that another of your children will have ADHD increases to about 33%. If you happen to be the parent of monozygotic ("identical") twins, the chance that the twin of a child diagnosed with ADHD increases to 75%.

What Is Inherited?

Multiple types of genetic characteristics have been identified in patients with ADHD. The most commonly reported ones involve chromosomes that are responsible for creating dopamine and norepinephrine transporters and receptors. It has been proposed that children with ADHD have an atypically high number of dopamine and norepinephrine reuptake transporters and fewer receptors for these neurotransmitters. This is what is believed to cause the underarousal of the brain. Although there is considerable debate among scientists about the specific inherited characteristics present in patients with ADHD, the high rate of heritability of ADHD is not an issue of debate at this time.

What Does All This Mean?

ADHD is an inherited medical condition that appears to be primarily associated with an underarousal of the regions of the brain that regulate mood, control behavior, and help us pay attention. This underarousal seems to be related to structural differences in brain cells that use dopamine and norepinephrine to communicate. Patients with ADHD appear to have dopamine and norepinephrine pathways that allow too much neurotransmitter to be reabsorbed. As a result, an insufficient amount of neurotransmitter is received by nearby cells. Those medical treatments that have been found to be effective in the treatment of ADHD target these underlying problems to achieve significant improvement in patients with ADHD.

Why Use Medicines to Treat ADHD?

Medicines for ADHD represent the most common type of treatment for this condition. At present, the FDA has approved four types of medications: methylphenidate-based medications (e.g., Ritalin, Concerta, Focalin, and Metadate), amphetamine-based medications (e.g., Dexedrine, Adderall, and Vyvanse), antihypertensive medications (e.g., clonidine, guanfacine, and Intuniv), and norepinephrine-specific reuptake inhibitors (atomoxetine [Strattera]). Some children and teens will present with sufficiently severe anxiety or anger-control problems that their physicians will combine ADHD medications with mood stabilizers (e.g., Abilify), anticonvulsant medications (e.g., Depakote), or antidepressant medications (e.g., Celexa, Zoloft, Paxil). At our clinic, we have found that such medications are rarely needed when careful attention is given to addressing sleep problems, dietary problems, and other medical and neurological conditions that can cause significant mood problems (e.g., vitamin D deficiencies).

ADHD medicines work in several ways. Some block the action of the *dopamine reuptake system* (e.g., methylphenidate, Ritalin, Concerta, Metadate, Focalin), which allows more dopamine to activate nearby brain cells. Other medications (e.g., Dexedrine) stimulate the release of dopamine, resulting in increased levels of this neurotransmitter at receptor sites. A third type of stimulant (Adderall, Vyvanse) stimulates the release of dopamine and norepinephrine and blocks the reuptake of these neurotransmitters. Nonstimulant ADHD medications, such as Strattera, primarily block the action of the norepinephrine reuptake system, which enhances the transmission neural pathways that use this neurotransmitter. Antihypertensive medications (e.g., clonidine, guanfacine, Intuniv) occupy adrenalin receptors and slow down the activation of neural pathways that can cause hyperarousal of the frontal lobes, as well as increased aggression and anxiety. If a patient is consuming an adequate amount of dietary protein, getting sufficient sleep, and does not have another medical condition that is causing ADHD-like symptoms, these medications are typically well tolerated. However, the benefits among patients who do not eat protein at breakfast and lunch appear to be reduced and the frequency of side effects (e.g., headaches, insomnia, stomachaches, irritability) is increased.

PSYCHOLOGICAL AND EDUCATIONAL TREATMENTS FOR ADHD

The consensus among health care professionals is that patients with ADHD are more successful at home, school, and in the community if their treatment includes a combination of medication and other types of interventions. Several types of treatments have been shown to yield positive results in both case studies and controlled group studies. These include

- the development of a program of academic support and accommodation at school;
- parenting classes to teach strategies that systematically use reinforcement to help children and adolescents develop essential life skills;
- social skills classes that help kids learn how to start and maintain conversations, establish friendships, resolve conflicts, and build self-confidence;
- electroencephalography biofeedback (also called *neurotherapy*), which promotes the development of attention and behavioral control by helping patients learn how to regulate the level of "arousal" in the regions of the brain that control these functions; and
- individual and family therapy to address problems of trauma, attachment disorders, inadequate parental nurturance, and excessive parent–child and marital conflict in the home.

Although I take a little time to describe each of these treatments, this book does not concentrate on how others can help your child. The purpose of this book is to help *you* learn ways to promote your child's success. The lessons to be shared involve learning about medication, nutrition, the educational rights of your child, and parenting approaches that can help your child mature. Although your parenting style did not cause ADHD, there is much that you can do to help.

HOMEWORK

Parents have numerous concerns when it comes to their child's development. This week, I'd like you to look at the list of lessons that you might want your child to learn (found at the end of this lesson).

Check off those that you'd like to teach your child. As you learn how to help your child develop skills, use this as a reference. Try not to get discouraged if you find yourself checking off 30 or 40 problems. Later in this book, I'll suggest that you focus on about a half dozen of your most pressing concerns, just to help you get comfortable. Once the techniques described in this book become part of your family life, it is a lot easier to address other problem areas.

After you pick out the lessons that you want to teach, I'd like you to consider establishing the Parent–Child Nonaggression Pact.

THE PARENT–CHILD NONAGGRESSION PACT

Change is not readily accepted in any organization, and families that include a patient diagnosed with ADHD are no exception. In addition, children and teens with ADHD are highly reactive to change in their environment and are likely to become verbally or physically aggressive when they don't get their way. To set the stage for teaching lessons, it helps to establish a Parent–Child Nonaggression Pact. The first part of this family rule is simply this: *It is not OK for anyone in the family to yell, threaten, hit, tease, or be mean to another family member.* That is not to say that it won't happen. Let's face it, at times you'll get angry and your child will get angry. Most likely, there will be moments when mean words are spoken. When that happens, I'd like you to consider instituting the second part of the Parent–Child Nonaggression Pact: *If a family member says or does something that is hurtful, when her or she cools off, that family member will apologize and do something to make up. That goes for everyone.*

In life, when we do (or say) something to another person that is hurtful, we owe that person an apology. It's also a good idea to try to make amends. I want my patients to learn that their parents are people and that it is important to be sensitive to the needs and feelings of others. So if they yell at their parents for 15 minutes, stomp around the living room, and slam doors just because they had to stop playing some video or computer game, that is not OK. Before they can resume playing anything, they will need to apologize and do something to make amends (e.g., do an extra chore, write a note describing what they should do instead of yelling, list why mom or dad deserves to be respected, write a noted describing what they like about mom or dad, make a snack for the family). I often say to my patients that if you make someone's life harder, you need to apologize and do something to make it better. So before you begin the next lesson, pick a calm moment, sit down with your child, explain this new family rule, and try it out.

When I offer this suggestion in my parenting classes, I have often heard parents wonder why I wouldn't encourage them to simply ground the child from use of their video-game system for a day or a week, instead of this make-up stuff. Certainly, that makes sense for a lot of kids. However, children with ADHD tend to blow up more intensely when you take away their stuff, sneak behind your back and play with the forbidden item anyway (hey, you're not there all the time), or simply start playing with one of the other electronic pleasure boxes available in most homes (e.g., phone, television, computer). I realize that you could hide the game, disconnect the electricity, and create an armed camp in your home. But to be honest, your child is probably going to relish that battle and lose sight of what you are actually trying to teach.

Despite such problems, I have no doubt that an energetic, determined, and forceful parent could pull off such takeaway strategies. However, as I explain to parents, I'm thinking of the long term. I'd like your child to develop the habit of offering an apology and attempting to make it up as early in life as possible. In healthy adult relationships, we don't take something away from our friend or spouse if they upset us or we upset them. Not if we want an enduring relationship. Instead, we offer an apology and attempt to make up. Why not teach *that* to your child?

What I'd Like My Child to Learn

1. _____ Wake up in the morning without battling with me
2. _____ Get dressed in clean clothes in the morning
3. _____ Eat breakfast that includes some kind of protein
4. _____ Take medication
5. _____ Brush teeth, wash up, comb hair
6. _____ Make bed, pick up room in the morning
7. _____ Pack school bag with books, homework, etc.
8. _____ Not argue with family members in the morning
9. _____ Get to the school bus on time
10. _____ Get to classes on time
11. _____ Remember to bring the necessary books and materials to class
12. _____ Remember to turn in homework
13. _____ Sit in seat at school
14. _____ Do school work in class
15. _____ Speak when called on in class
16. _____ Not interrupt the teacher
17. _____ Eat a healthy lunch
18. _____ Copy down homework assignments
19. _____ Remember to bring home the books and materials needed for homework
20. _____ Learn how to have conversations with other kids
21. _____ Learn how to play and solve disagreements without getting into fights
22. _____ Come home after school
23. _____ Do homework
24. _____ Organize books and school materials so that work doesn't get lost
25. _____ Listen and obey parental instructions
26. _____ Come home for dinner
27. _____ Eat a dinner that includes protein, fruit, and vegetables
28. _____ Do chores with minimal prompting
29. _____ Play cooperatively with siblings and friends
30. _____ Put away toys, papers, etc.

(continued)

What I'd Like My Child to Learn (*Continued*)

31. _____ Clean room
32. _____ Not argue with parents
33. _____ Learn to solve problems by negotiating
34. _____ Spend some time reading, painting, building, practicing word-processing skills, or engaging in any activity that requires thinking
35. _____ Express ideas or feelings without using obscene or vulgar language
36. _____ Wash up, brush teeth in the evening
37. _____ Go to the bedroom at bedtime and rest quietly
38. _____ Stay in the bedroom and let me sleep until morning
39. _____ Apologize, accept responsibility for mistakes, and make up
40. _____ Do something thoughtful for another person

Other Lessons? _____

© Vincent J. Monastra, PhD

MEDICINES DON'T CURE ADHD, BUT THEY CAN HELP

One of the most hotly debated topics in the United States centers on the use of medications in treating childhood psychiatric disorders such as attention-deficit/hyperactivity disorder (ADHD). At one extreme are advocates of medication who assert that these medicines are effective and absolutely safe for children. These individuals point to the decades of use of stimulant therapy, to double-blind studies that show short-term improvement of attention and reduction of hyperactivity and impulsivity, and to the absence of any medical evidence showing that the use of these medications causes harm to patients. The poster child for this advocacy group is the kid who was inattentive, out of control, and flunking out of school before using medication. After using medication, this same child is maintaining a degree of organization that would make Martha Stewart proud and is a straight-*A* student.

At the other extreme are parents and health care professionals who are alarmed that doctors are prescribing stimulant medications to children and teens. These individuals express concern about increasing the risk for substance abuse in children with ADHD, cite evidence that suggests chronic use of amphetamines may alter brain structures, and assert that medicines for ADHD simply put more money in the pockets of drug companies and doctors and make energetic kids more manageable for lazy parents and teachers. The poster child for this advocacy group is the child who became a zombie, reacted with increased aggression or hyperactivity, or started hallucinating after taking a stimulant medication.

SO WHO'S TELLING THE TRUTH?

From my perspective, both sides are telling the truth. One thing I've learned in my clinical work is to listen to my patients and their parents. As a psychologist who has participated in the evaluation and treatment of at least 15,000 patients diagnosed with ADHD and other behavioral disorders, I have seen the poster children from both advocacy groups. There is substantial evidence from research studies and clinical practice that medications for ADHD can improve attention and behavioral control. They can also help patients control commonly occurring emotional problems such as anxiety, depressed mood, and outbursts of temper. If a patient is diagnosed on the basis of a thorough evaluation process (that includes screening for other relevant medical conditions), receives a dose of medication that has been properly adjusted, is getting sufficient sleep, and is eating something more substantial than cereal for breakfast and chips and soda for lunch, then medications like Adderall-XR, Concerta, Focalin-XR, Metadate-CD, and others can be helpful.

However, if the diagnosis is based on a cursory interview or a knee-jerk reaction to parent or teacher complaints, if dosage is based on age or body weight, and if no attention is paid to a child's dietary and sleep habits, these medications can cause substantial short-term problems. I have seen many kids in my office who were responding poorly to stimulants. The typical parent story goes something like this.

Timmy has been having a hard time sitting still in school ever since kindergarten. His teacher thought that he was just an energetic, bright student and understood that he needed to be able to move around in class. Things went OK that year, but this year his teacher insisted that he stay in his chair and do his class work. Timmy kept getting up and talking with other kids and got angry when his teacher told him to sit down. One day, it got really bad, and he pushed his chair at his teacher. She called us and told us that she thought he might have ADHD.

So we took Timmy to see his pediatrician. The doctor spoke with us for 10 minutes and asked us to complete a form that asked a lot of questions about our son's ability to listen, follow directions, and things like that. The doctor also asked us to give the teacher a form for her to fill out. After the forms were completed, we saw the doctor again, and were told that Timmy has ADHD. The doctor spoke with us about stimulant medications, and we decided to try a medication that lasted all day. Because our son was only 7 years old, the doctor suggested that we start with Concerta (18 mg).

The first day, Timmy wasn't hungry for breakfast, which wasn't unusual. But we gave him the medication. He went off to school and his teacher told us that she thought he had a pretty good day. He stayed in his seat, seemed to pay attention, and didn't get angry. Timmy complained that his stomach felt upset a little and his head hurt, but this went away. But he didn't eat much lunch either. That night, Timmy was off the wall. He ran around in circles, yelling and screaming, and wore himself out by 9:00 p.m.

The next day, we still couldn't get any breakfast into Timmy. He took his medication and went to school. That day wasn't as good as the day before, but his teacher still said she thought the medication was helping. After school, we couldn't see any improvement, and as the night wore on, Timmy revved up. We decided to call the pediatrician.

The doctor told us that this was common. He suggested that we increase the dose to 36 mg of Concerta so that the medicine would work longer. We did. The next day, his teacher told us he was refusing to do his schoolwork. We told Timmy that he couldn't go outside to play. He blew up and trashed his room. Later on, he calmed down a little bit, but that night, he didn't fall asleep until 11:00 p.m. I didn't know what to do. I called his doctor the next day.

The doctor told me that some kids start to adjust to their medication after a little while. I was told to keep him on that dose for the rest of the month and to come in for an appointment. That month was hell. My son ate like a bird, was fighting with me and my husband all the time, and refused to do anything at school. When we saw the doctor, we decided to increase his medication to 54 mg of Concerta.

Not much changed for the better after that. Timmy still wouldn't eat, was moody and angry, and got into trouble at school nearly every day. At the end of the month, his doctor said that perhaps we should try a different stimulant. We changed to Adderall-XR (20 mg). Still no change. His doctor said that maybe something else was wrong with Timmy. He suggested that we consult with a psychiatrist or psychologist. We decided to see you because you specialize in treating kids with ADHD.

So what went wrong? There are several possibilities. First, Timmy's doctor did not test to see if there was any other medical explanation for his symptoms. In addition, there was no evaluation of the adequacy of his diet and no examination of sleeping patterns. Although I reviewed the importance of diet, adequate sleep, and a thorough medical evaluation in Lesson 2, these factors cannot be overemphasized if you want your child to succeed.

There is one other explanation for Timmy's poor response to medication: the presence of another neurological condition that is causing his symptoms. During the past 25 years, nearly a dozen research teams have examined thousands of patients with ADHD and found that the vast majority (80%–90%) demonstrated under-activity in the frontal lobes of the brain. However, there is a *neurophysiological subgroup* of patients with ADHD who do not show such cortical slowing.

One of the first researchers who identified this subgroup was Dr. Daniel Amen, using single-photon emission computed tomography (SPECT) imaging. Unlike other patients with ADHD, this group demonstrated excessive "fast" electroencephalogram activity, particularly in a region called the cingulate gyrus. Children with hyperarousal in the cingulate gyrus and who do not show excessive slowing in the frontal lobes typically come for treatment because of a combination of attention, anxiety, mood, or anger-control problems. Like our research team, Dr. Amen's group found that methylphenidate-based medications, such as Concerta or Focalin-XR, are rarely helpful with these patients. He has described a number of useful strategies for treating this group in various books and professional publications. You can find information about Dr. Amen's use of SPECT imaging and treatment online (Amen Clinics; see www.amenclinics.com).

Other research teams using quantitative electroencephalography (QEEG) procedures have also found evidence of excessive activity in a subgroup of patients with ADHD (about 10%–20%). By measuring the electrical activity in the brains of children and teens as they perform academic tasks, researchers have found that those children who do not demonstrate underactivity of the brain typically do not respond to methylphenidate-based medications. This makes a lot of sense when we start to look more closely at those patients who do not respond positively to methylphenidate-based medications.

For example, we know that a substantial percentage of patients with ADHD (15%–35%) will either not respond positively to such stimulant medication or will be unable to tolerate side effects. When such patients have been examined with QEEG, it is frequently found that they do not demonstrate cortical slowing. Consequently, it is not surprising that they would not respond to medications designed to stimulate increased brain activation in the frontal lobes (which is the result of using methylphenidate). After all, if a patient's brain is not working too slowly, then why should we expect a stimulant medication like Concerta to help?

Because of this research, one of the tests I routinely use in my evaluation of patients who have attention problems or display hyperactivity-impulsivity is a QEEG examination. I have found that this is particularly helpful in situations in which the child has responded poorly to stimulant medications, when there is skepticism about the medical "reality" of the child's attention problems, and when parents are uncomfortable with the idea of using medication for ADHD. As one dad put it, "If ADHD is a medical condition, then there should be some sort of physical sign."

In 2013, the U.S. Food and Drug Administration (FDA) agreed that QEEG technology provided such a sign and approved a QEEG test based on the process developed and patented by myself and Dr. Joel Lubar for use in the diagnosis of ADHD. Parents interested in learning more about the development of this test can visit the FDA's website (www.fda.gov/newsevents/newsroom/pressannouncements/ucm360811.htm or www.accessdata.fda.gov/cdrh_docs/pdf), the Biofeedback Federation of Europe's website (www.bfe.org), or read the discussion about this test on Medscape (www.medscape.com/viewarticle/809079).

The concept behind this test is relatively straightforward. As I tell the parents and children I evaluate,

> The brain has a beat, just like your heart. And, just like your heart, the harder it is working, the faster it beats. We've learned that when the brain beats too slowly, we have a hard time paying attention and staying still. We also learned that the brain beating too fast can also be a problem. That's true for our hearts, too. So today, we'll place some little stethoscopes on the top of your head and check out how fast your brain is pulsing.

I then show the child pictures about what the pulse of the brain looks like, and within 10 to 20 minutes we're ready to begin. Depending on the type of QEEG evaluation process used, the test takes 20 to 30 minutes to administer.

The process is painless, and nearly all of the children I've worked with are fascinated by watching the pulse of their brain. However, I've found that children with tactile sensitivities often need to touch the sensors and watch me place them on their parents. Sometimes, I'll ask parents to assist me in placing sensors, if their child is especially uncomfortable with being touched by a stranger. In the thousands of patients of evaluated, only once have I been unable to complete this procedure, and that child returned to the clinic another day and handled the process well. The results of this type of examination are easily translated to children, parents, and teachers; they help all involved better understand the physical foundations of ADHD, support the establishment of appropriate medical and educational interventions, and reduce the chance that your child will have a poor medication response. If you happen to live in an area where this type of QEEG examination is available, I suggest you consider including it in your child's evaluation. The Association for Applied Psychophysiology and Biofeedback (www.aapb.org; 303-422-8546) or the International Society for Neurofeedback and Research (www.isnr.org; phone: 800-488-3867) can provide a listing of providers in your region who are qualified to complete such an evaluation.

DO ALL KIDS NEED STIMULANTS?

No. One thing that I want to cover in this lesson is the different types of medications used to treat patients with ADHD. Depending on the kinds of symptoms, some children will be treated with methylphenidate-based stimulants (e.g., Concerta, Focalin-XR), some with amphetamine-based stimulants (e.g., Adderall-XR, Vyvanse), some with nonstimulant ADHD medications (e.g., Strattera), and some with antihypertensive medications (e.g., Catapres, Tenex, Intuniv). Other types of medications include stimulatory antidepressants (e.g., Wellbutrin), anticonvulsants (e.g., Depakote, Tegretol), and selective serotonin reuptake inhibitor (SSRI) antidepressants. I'll spend the rest of this lesson describing how each can be used to promote your child's success.

MEDICINES FOR PROBLEMS OF INATTENTION, HYPERACTIVITY, AND IMPULSIVITY

The primary type of treatment for the core symptoms of ADHD (inattention, impulsivity, and hyperactivity) is stimulant medication. As I described in Lesson 2, these medications help to increase the activity of the brain by stimulating brain cells to fire more rapidly by blocking the cells' ability to reabsorb specific neurotransmitters or by causing both of these changes. For example, when a person takes a medication like Dexedrine, brain cells that communicate by releasing dopamine are stimulated to increase their activity. Presumably, the increased availability of dopamine serves to help the communication between brain cells responsible for attention and behavioral control.

In a similar manner, other medications (e.g., Ritalin, methylphenidate, Concerta, Metadate-CD, Focalin-XR) try to boost the communication of dopamine-bearing brain cells by occupying the dopamine reuptake transporter system. When brain cells release a bit of their neurotransmitter, the dopamine reuptake transport system tries to recapture some of this brain "juice" so that the cell can send another message. Medicines like Ritalin (and related compounds) attach to these reuptake transporters, preventing them from "capturing" dopamine. In doing so, dopamine remains in the space between the brain cells (called a synapse) for a longer period of time and can activate nearby brain cells more intensely. In the case of dopamine-bearing brain cells, the result can be improved attention, concentration, and behavioral control.

The last type of stimulant medication commonly available is called Adderall (the longer acting version is called Adderall-XR). This medication is approximately twice as potent as Ritalin. That means 5 mg of Adderall has about the same effect as a 10-mg dose of Ritalin. The reason for this is the dual action of Adderall. Like Dexedrine, this medication increases the release of dopamine from brain cells. In addition, like Ritalin, this medication blocks the ability of the dopamine reuptake transport system to reabsorb dopamine after it has been released from a brain cell. Adderall also stimulates the release and blocks the reuptake of norepinephrine, another neurotransmitter involved in helping us sustain attention and concentrate.

So when your child begins to take a methylphenidate-based medication, the physician is attempting to treat his or her medical condition by increasing the level of dopamine that is available to help brain cells communicate. This increased dopamine activity occurs in regions of the brain responsible for attention and concentration (generally the frontal lobes), in brain structures involved in mood regulation (primarily the thalamus and limbic system), and in neurological centers responsible for planned movement (the rolandic cortex). When doctors prescribe an amphetamine-based stimulant, they are attempting to treat the condition by increasing the levels of norepinephrine and dopamine. In doing so, doctors are using a medication that also improves the activation of the cerebellum, a brain region involved in social judgment and planning. Although dopamine- and norepinephrine-bearing brain cells do not carry out these jobs alone (there are numerous other brain chemicals that can be involved), medications that target these systems can have a profound effect in improving a child's attention and behavior.

Start-Up Strategies

If a parent is comfortable with the use of medication for ADHD, the next step is to identify an optimal type and dose of medication. To figure this out, collaboration among the child's physician, parents, teachers, and psychologist or other mental health specialist is needed. Typically, a physician will prescribe the lowest dose available for a particular type of medication—for example, 18 mg of Concerta, 20 mg of Metadate-CD, or the equivalent of this in other stimulants (e.g., 5 mg of Adderall-XR). Parents and teachers would be asked to provide information about how well the medication is working and if any side effects are occurring. At our clinic, we use the Medication Response Chart and the Medication Tolerance Checklist to help us get a better idea of how a medication is working (samples are provided at the end of this lesson).

These types of questionnaires can be helpful in adjusting the amount of medication needed. For example, although medications are supposed to last a certain amount of time, a child's actual response may be quite different. I have treated children who are using Concerta (a medication that can provide symptomatic relief for 10–12 hours) and show poor attention and become hyperactive after 6 hours. Similarly, I have seen children who are being treated with Adderall-XR (which can provide 10–12 hours of clinical improvement) show problems with attention, behavioral control, or moodiness in the late afternoon or early evening. If your child is taking one of these medications but her or his teacher is saying it isn't working, try to track down when the medicine seems to be wearing off.

Sometimes, what's needed is a higher dose of medication in the morning or an early-afternoon booster of a low dose of an immediate release type of stimulant (e.g., adding Ritalin or Adderall between noon and 3 p.m.). At other times, combining a stimulant with other medications (e.g., antihypertensives like Catapres or Tenex or a nonstimulant ADHD medication like Strattera) can help to reduce hyperactivity and moodiness after school without causing disruption of eating or sleeping habits. I will typically repeat a computerized test of attention and conduct QEEG examination at the time when the medication effects seem to be wearing off to obtain a physical measure of the attention loss.

In other instances, a child can show problems during the later part of the school day or at home not because of the ineffectiveness of medication but because of an underlying learning disorder or because they are being asked to complete tasks that are commonly difficult for children with ADHD (e.g., writing, repetitive copying, note taking, text reading). In those instances, provision of word-processing tools, voice-recognition software (e.g., Dragon's Naturally Speaking), or text-reading software (e.g., Kurzweil, Read & Write: Gold Edition) can be helpful. Free versions of voice-recognition and text-reading software are also available (e.g., Panopreter Basic, Ultra Hal Text-to-Read Speech Reader). A helpful website that can guide you in your search for software to help your child complete reading and writing tasks can be found at www.howtogeek.com.

The deterioration of medication effects is not limited to the school day and the performance of academic tasks. However, it sometimes surprises me that parents get the impression that they should just tough it out once their children get home. I consider success at home to be just as important for a child's development as success at school. If a child goes home every day and begins to get yelled at, ignored, criticized, hit, grounded, or punished by having their favorite activities taken away from them because they don't listen, play quietly, not interrupt, for example, then the child is not going to be feeling loved and cared about. Rather, the child is going to be feeling miserable—and acting miserably as well (and so will you).

Because of this, I also track how the child is doing after school. I consider medication to be somewhat like a knee brace used after a joint injury. It doesn't cure the medical problem, but it helps a person get around and live their life. As I'm one of those weekend warriors with chronic knee and ankle injuries, I need to be careful. If I'm going to be physically active in the morning, I need to tape and use a brace. If I'm going to be physically active in the afternoon, I need to tape and use a brace. And guess what? If I'm playing softball after work, I need to tape and use a brace. If I don't, then my ankle is going to give out, and that's not fun. So if I'm a kid who uses medication to help me pay attention, concentrate, and control my reactions to frustration during the day, then the odds are I'll need to be treated with some type of medication that can help me succeed at home and on the ball field or dance studio in the evening.

I often hear that parents and physicians are reluctant to prescribe medications that will remain clinically active in the afternoon and early evening, because of concerns about sleeping problems. It is well known that kids who use stimulants can have a hard time getting to sleep at night. As a result, parents and physicians have been reluctant to prescribe stimulant medication that can help in the late afternoon and early evening. Although I respect this caution, I think there are other interventions that can be used, rather than taking a child's medication away for the last 4 waking hours.

For example, I do not ignore the importance of dietary issues at my clinic. I often ask about what a child is eating during the day. It is far from uncommon to find that a child who can't fall asleep eats little protein during the day, consumes all sorts of energizing carbohydrates that combine sugars and chocolate, drinks caffeinated beverages, and, because of parent work schedules and after-school activities, eats his or her largest meal between 6:00 and 7:00 p.m. By not eating protein until the late afternoon or early evening, they are depriving their bodies of the raw material (the amino acid tryptophan) that is necessary to make melatonin, which is the chemical that puts us to sleep. Consequently, I try to help parents find ways to improve their child's intake of protein at breakfast and lunch and eat dinner earlier so that the late afternoon and early evening hours can be more positive times for them and their children (more on that in the next lesson).

In addition to focusing on the child's diet, I also ask about the child's activities in the evening. An increasing number of children spend much of their evening fixated on bright, highly stimulatory video screens, positioned about 18 to 24 inches from their eyes. Because exposure to bright light inhibits the production of melatonin (and delays sleep), I encourage parents to discontinue this kind of activity at least 1.5 hours before bedtime. I'm also a big fan of my patient's involvement in any type of full-body activity that gives a good cardiovascular workout at some time in the day (e.g., swimming, biking, dancing, drumming, hiking, hockey, basketball, football). My little guys are asleep within nanoseconds on days that we spend an hour or so at a pool or bike around a park. On days when they're little coach potatoes, bedtime can drag on forever.

How Do I Know That the Dose Is the Right One?

The process for determining type and dose of medication is not a matter of simply starting a medication, asking parents and teachers if it is generally working, and then increasing dose or changing the type of medication. It requires doctors to look closely at when medication is "working" or "not working"; finding out what the child is being asked to do when difficulties are noted; discovering which strategies parents and teachers use at those times to encourage effort; monitoring the child's dietary, exercise, and sleeping habits; and testing the child's attention at those times when problems are occurring. On the basis of test results and parent and teacher information, changes in the treatment plan can be introduced. Sometimes providing academic support at school is needed. Sometimes making changes in the child's diet, sleep schedule, and activities is required. Other times, decreasing the time between doses, increasing dose, or adding an additional dose(s) is what is necessary. Typically, introducing a motivational program at home and school is also needed. Let's play out a couple of scenarios. Keep in mind that in each of these illustrations, the child has been thoroughly evaluated by his or her physician for other medical problems that could cause symptoms of inattention, hyperactivity, and impulsivity.

The first scenario reflects a pattern I have seen frequently. It is one in which a child, let's say an 8-year-old, starts taking a medication such as Concerta (18 mg). The teacher reports that the child's behavior is improving but that he is still having difficulties remaining seated and staying quiet and on task during the day. His parents tell me that after school there is no change. It's like their child isn't even taking medication. Because psychologists and other health care providers now have reliable, computerized tests to measure attention (e.g., continuous performance tests such as the IVA, TOVA, or Conners' Continuous Performance Test) and QEEG tests can provide a physiological indicator of the child's attention at any time of day, I use information from these kinds of tests in my evaluation of medication effects. In the situation I'm describing here, the results of a computerized test of attention (the IVA) that was administered 2 hours after taking Concerta in the morning indicated that the child's performance on that test had improved since starting medication and was now consistent with his age group. That finding was consistent with the teacher report that the child seemed "better." However, the Medication Response Chart the teacher completed also indicated that by lunchtime, the child was really struggling to maintain attention and behavioral control. What would I recommend?

First, I'd want to make sure that the child's dietary patterns included consumption of protein-based foods throughout the day (approximately 10–15 grams at each meal, based on U.S. Department of Agriculture recommendations for an 8-year-old). Why? Because the child is showing deterioration of functioning during the school day and little improvement at home, and such symptoms can occur when a child is not eating sufficient protein. So I'd want to make sure that the child is consuming the kinds of foods that can be used to make dopamine, norepinephrine, and serotonin (a neurotransmitter involved in mood regulation and sleep). After the child's protein intake has improved, I'd ask the teacher to complete a Medication Response Chart for 3 to 5 days to find out if and when the child is still showing deterioration of medication effects.

If the child was still struggling to stay focused and in control despite improving diet, I'd identify the times of day that are most problematic and repeat the QEEG examination at these challenging times. Although such testing does require taking your child out of school, this kind of information provides an indicator of how physically alert and attentive your son or daughter is and helps to clarify whether medical factors (rather than motivational or learning problems) are at the root of your child's continued difficulties during the school day. I'd also find out what types of activities are occurring during these challenging times. It is not unusual for symptoms to increase during academic tasks that are particularly difficult for the child (e.g., doing mathematics problems, completing writing assignments).

If QEEG findings indicated that the child was demonstrating abnormal brain activation patterns during challenging academic periods, despite medication, I would discuss adjusting medication with the child's physician (either increasing dose or considering an alternate stimulant). I'd continue this process until EEG indicators of attention revealed that the child's brain activation patterns were within age expectations. Once the child was demonstrating age-appropriate levels of brain activation, I'd check with the teacher to see if any learning or educational performance problems were persisting. If problems were continuing, I'd initially ask the teacher to see what happens if the child is given a bit more support in the classroom (e.g., seating close to the teacher, pairing with positive peers). If this is insufficient (and the child has not been referred to the school district's committee on special education), I would encourage his parents to request an evaluation by this committee so that the functional impact of the child's health impairment (i.e., ADHD) could be identified by the school district and an Instructional Support Plan, Accommodation Plan, or Individual Education Plan could be developed, depending on need. I discuss this process more fully in Lesson 5.

Another common situation occurs when the child shows positive response during the school day but loses focus and demonstrates behavioral control problems after school. If that is the case, then I would conduct a QEEG or administer the IVA or TOVA after school. If abnormal patterns of activation were evident at that time, then a low dose of a short-acting stimulant like Ritalin could be considered after school. Another option would consist of administration of a booster dose of a stimulant with 6 to 8 hours of benefits after lunch (e.g., Focalin, Adderall). If such an intervention causes difficulties falling asleep, antihypertensive medications such as Catapres or Tenex could be considered. Melatonin supplements (1–3 mg, administered 1.5–2.0 hours before bedtime) could be considered.

In both of these examples, a combination of parent and teacher observations, computerized tests of attention, and a QEEG examination is considered in guiding medication selection and adjustment. As I reported in a 2005 study of more than 1,500 patients, use of this type of approach leads to a marked improvement in treatment initiation and response rates. Although a provider able to perform all three of these types of evaluations may not be available in your community at this time, the FDA approval of QEEG assessment for ADHD should result in improved access to this type of testing in the near future.

What Happens If My Child Does Not Respond or Can't Tolerate Stimulants?

About a third of children with ADHD either do not respond to methylphenidate (the active ingredient in Ritalin, Concerta, Focalin, and Metadate-CD) or cannot tolerate this type of medication because of side effects. When the issue is one of insufficient response, it is common to try a more potent stimulant (e.g., Adderall-XR or Vyvanse). When the issue is that of inability to tolerate the medication (e.g., because of dramatic loss of appetite, severe sleep disturbance, or development of muscular blinks or spasms called *tics*), other medications may prove helpful. These include norepinephrine specific reuptake inhibitors (e.g., Strattera), stimulatory antidepressants (e.g., Wellbutrin, Effexor, Imipramine), antihypertensives (e.g., Catapres, Tenex, Intuniv), and anticonvulsant medications (e.g., Depakote, Tegretol).

Among those patients who are diagnosed with ADHD but do not show cortical slowing during QEEG examination, many demonstrate a positive response to combinations of antihypertensives such as Catapres, Tenex, or Intuniv and low doses of mixed amphetamine salts (e.g., Adderall, Adderall-XR, Vyvanse). A smaller percentage will respond to combinations of mixed amphetamine salts and SSRI-type antidepressants (e.g., Zoloft, Paxil, Celexa, Lexapro). Highly aggressive patients who do not respond to antihypertensives are sometimes treated by their physicians or psychiatrists with mood stabilizers or anticonvulsants in combination with Adderall-XR. However, such children typically have other medical conditions contributing to their attention problems (e.g., sleep disorders, nutritional deficiencies). Here is how these medications work.

Norepinephrine-specific reuptake inhibitors attempt to increase brain activity by inhibiting the reabsorption of the neurotransmitter norepinephrine. Because neural pathways that use norepinephrine also activate those brain regions involved in attention, concentration, behavioral control, and social judgment, medications (like Strattera) that enhance the functioning of norepinephrine pathways can also reduce the core symptoms of ADHD. This type of medication was developed primarily because of the number of patients who do not respond to stimulant therapy, cannot be treated with stimulants because of tics, who develop marked appetite suppression and weight loss with stimulants, and because of parent concerns about the potential abuse of these medications. My experience with Strattera is that although it can be helpful in improving attention, it needs to be combined with other medications (e.g., antihypertensives) in treating symptoms of hyperactivity-impulsivity. I have also found that Strattera can be sedating when given to a child in the morning, and I encourage parents whose children use this medication to introduce it at lunchtime or later in the afternoon.

Stimulatory antidepressant medications (e.g., Wellbutrin, Effexor, Imipramine) can be useful in treating patients whose primary ADHD symptoms are inattentive in nature. These medications facilitate the activity of several neurological pathways (including dopamine and norepinephrine ones) that are involved in attention and mood control. They can enhance attention and also help by reducing some of the irritability commonly shown by children with ADHD. However, these medications need to be administered for a month or so before you begin to see improvement in your child. Because parents (and their children) hope for more immediate benefits, these medications are typically prescribed when a child is unable to tolerate stimulants or if other medical problems (e.g., bedwetting) are a significant concern. Medications such as imipramine can be used in treating enuresis and ADHD and are often helpful in my younger patients.

Antihypertensive medications (Catapres, Tenex, Intuniv) are essentially medications that control blood pressure and can help ADHD patients by reducing symptoms of hyperactivity and impulsivity. They work by occupying brain receptors that are sensitive to adrenaline. Patients with high blood pressure take higher doses of these medications to reduce the risk of heart attack that comes with stress. During stressful moments, adrenaline is released by the adrenal glands, causing a variety of physical changes, including increased heart rate and blood pressure. Medications such as Catapres, Tenex, and Intuniv moderate the effect of adrenaline, keeping heart rate and blood pressure stable. When taken in low doses by patients with ADHD, these medications can reduce hyperactivity. In patients who demonstrate excessive activation of the brain on QEEG examination, these medications can also help to "slow down" the overly active brain and improve attention. We've found that Catapres seems particularly useful in the treatment of aggressive outbursts in children and teens with ADHD. Tenex seems more helpful when treating the anxiety and obsessive–compulsive–like symptoms that can occur in ADHD patients. Intuniv is simply an extended-release version of Tenex (lasting about 10–12 hours). Patients who demonstrate cortical slowing on QEEG will show more severe symptoms of inattention if treated with antihypertensives alone (because these medications slow down the brain).

Anticonvulsant medications (e.g., Tegretol and Depakote) were initially developed to control seizures. Clinical research has indicated that these medications can also treat symptoms of hyperactivity and aggression in children with ADHD who do not respond to stimulant medications. However, because anticonvulsant medications do not typically improve attention, tend to suppress intellectual functions, and can adversely affect liver function, they are rarely a first-line treatment for ADHD.

SSRI-type antidepressants (Zoloft, Paxil, Lexapro, Celexa) can also be used in the treatment of ADHD patients who do not respond or are unable to tolerate stimulants. Patients diagnosed with ADHD but who do not show cortical slowing on QEEG examination have shown improvement in attention, mood, and behavioral control after treatment with this type of medication. These medicines work by enhancing the activity of brain cells that use the neurotransmitter serotonin. Descriptively, neural pathways that use serotonin appear to exert a primary effect on mood. In research efforts, I have found that Zoloft appears particularly useful for patients with ADHD who tend to lose their temper frequently; Paxil and Celexa seem to help ADHD patients who are anxious; Lexapro seems beneficial with symptoms of depression. However, caution is advised in the use of SSRIs because recent studies indicate that increased depression can occur when children and teens are treated with SSRIs and that withdrawal effects can be severe when these medications are discontinued. Consequently, this type of medication is one that we use at my clinic only when the patient does not respond to antihypertensives and I am certain that other medical conditions are not causing the child's problems.

Medications for Temper, Anxiety, and Depression

Children and teens with ADHD commonly have problems that go beyond inattention, hyperactivity, and impulsivity. Many of these patients struggle to control their temper, their worries, and their despair. Parents of children and teens with ADHD can be stunned by the intensity of their child's reactions to disappointment and frustration, alarmed by their child's extensive worries over seemingly nothing, and the degree of despair sometimes shown by these children. Kids with ADHD can become highly explosive when they don't get their way or when they are punished or face consequences of their actions. They can spend endless hours worrying about disease and disaster. They can talk about wishing they were dead or how they are going to jump out the window or kill everyone just because you won't take them to Burger King.

Why Does This Happen?

Big question. Little answer. The frontal lobes, as well as other regions of the brain (e.g., the cerebellum, which appears important for social judgment), appear essential in helping people control their emotional reactions. There is a tendency to think that the problems in "waking up" the part of the brain essential for attention and concentration are limited to forgetting homework and avoiding chores. They're not. The regions of the brain that are involved in paying attention in school and concentrating on your history homework are also involved in figuring out what to do and how to calm down when mom and dad say no or when your brother won't get off the computer. The difficulties a child with ADHD has in regulating the frontal lobes will contribute not only to problems learning at school but also to difficulties solving problems at home.

As a result, the medications that were described for treating ADHD also can have a beneficial effect on mood problems. Sometimes stimulants alone can help with these problems. Sometimes they need to be combined with other medications (typically antihypertensives, but antidepressants, anticonvulsants, or mood stabilizers may be used in severe situations). Regardless of the type of medication used, it is important to realize that these medications will help to tone down the emotional reaction. However, it will be up to you, as well as your child's teachers, counselors, and doctors, to teach your child how to effectively express his or her emotional reactions and solve problems in social situations. Much of this book concentrates on that process.

If you are a parent of a child who is talking about hurting him- or herself or is threatening to hurt you or others, you need to make sure that your child's physician, psychologist, or other mental health provider is aware of this—even if the child has not acted on his or her threats. Even though children and teens with ADHD are more likely to make dramatic statements when upset, it is not a good idea to ignore them. Sometimes increased emotionality can occur because of vitamin D deficiency or other medical problems. Sometimes it can be a side effect of medications. Sometimes what is needed is the inclusion of medication to specifically address mood problems. And sometimes what is needed is instruction in how to handle frustration. Regardless of the cause, when a child is talking about hurting him- or herself or others, it is important that this information be shared with someone who can help sort out the causes and provide appropriate care.

What If I Am Not Comfortable Using Any Type of Medication?

It is not uncommon for parents to be uncomfortable with the idea of giving their child a "brain medication." In fact, one of the primary reasons treatment of patients with ADHD is not initiated is because parents' concerns have not been sufficiently addressed by their doctor. I hope the information in this book will clarify some of the ways you can address your concerns about the use of medication.

However, many parents are interested in learning about how they can help improve their children's attention and behavioral control without medication. Their hope is that they can reduce the amount of medication needed or perhaps help their child overcome ADHD without needing to use medication. Since the last edition of this book was written, there have been substantial developments in research examining treatments for ADHD that do not include medication. Among the psychological treatments that have been studied, EEG biofeedback, computerized attention-training programs, social skills training, individual coaching, parent counseling, and family therapy have received the most interest.

Although each of these treatments appears to provide some benefit in promoting the social development of children with ADHD,

EEG biofeedback (also called *neurofeedback*) has sufficient scientific support to be considered an effective treatment for ADHD. A published *meta-analysis* (i.e., a study comparing the results of many published studies) of EEG biofeedback research indicated a large effect on symptoms of inattention and impulsivity and a medium effect on hyperactivity. Certain other computerized attention-training programs (e.g., CogMed, Captain's Log, and the online web-based training program Lumosity) also seem to contribute to improvements in attention. In addition, there are several apps available (e.g., through BanzaiLabs) that some kids find helpful. Other home-based biofeedback devices (e.g., HeartMath) help children and teens learn how to control heart-rate variability and, in doing so, improve attention and emotional control.

Because of the significant improvements in attention, impulse control, and academic performance that have been reported in the scientific literature, there has been considerable interest in the use of EEG biofeedback for ADHD. Many of the parents who are interested in EEG biofeedback for their children have heard horror stories about children and teens who have experienced dramatic negative reactions to medication. Others worry about the long-term effects of stimulants, have fears that stimulants will turn their children into junkies, or have heard that medications do not always work. Perhaps they have mistakenly heard that EEG biofeedback cures all of the problems associated with ADHD. Perhaps they are just hoping that it helps a bit.

Regardless of the reasons parents are interested in EEG biofeedback, the scientific evidence reported to date clearly indicates that children, teens, and adults with ADHD who are treated with this method improve in a variety of ways. Patients have demonstrated significant changes on neurological indicators of brain functioning (functional magnetic resonance imaging, QEEG) and improvement on computerized tests of attention. Questionnaires completed by parents and teachers indicated significant improvement in the core symptoms of ADHD. Improved scores on tests of intelligence and scholastic abilities have also been reported when using this type of treatment. These improvements have been sustained in multiple well-controlled published studies in which children were randomly assigned to EEG biofeedback or other credible comparison interventions. In addition, follow-up examination of patients after EEG biofeedback treatment has indicated the gains from this treatment improvement is enduring. At this time, the American Academy of Pediatrics has concluded that EEG biofeedback has the best level of scientific support for the treatment of ADHD (which is the same level of support as medications for ADHD).

How Does EEG Biofeedback (Neurotherapy) Work?

The basic idea behind this therapy is that if a patient is able to learn how to control the level of brain activity in those regions that control attention and planned motor activity, then improvement of attention and reduction of hyperactivity should occur. Patients learn to improve by receiving information (called *feedback*) in the form of sounds and pictures that are shown on a computer monitor. Essentially, the patient receives a tone and watches video screen changes every time he or she produces the desired type of brain activity for one-half of a second. The patient's task is to learn how to produce more of these half-second alert periods. As patients do so, improvement in the core symptoms of ADHD have been show to occur, typically within 30 to 40 sessions.

Although clinical researchers continue to try to understand how this treatment specifically works and how long the improvements will remain, there is little scientific reason to doubt that clinical improvements typically occur in patients treated with this type of therapy. The primary limitation of this type of therapy is the short-term cost and the availability of providers. Although most insurance companies now recognize EEG biofeedback as a treatment for ADHD, which makes it a more feasible option for parents, many communities do not have qualified providers. To learn more about this type of treatment and providers in your community, you can contact the Biofeedback Certification International Alliance (www. bcia.org), the Association for Applied Psychophysiology and Biofeedback (www.aapb.org), or the International Society for Neurofeedback and Research (www.isnr.org).

What Can I Do If I Can't Find a Provider or Can't Afford EEG Biofeedback?

If you are interested in exploring the benefits of computerized training of attention and working memory at home, there are several options. CogMed and Captain's Log are computer programs that can be purchased for improving attention and working memory. These programs engage children in a series of tasks designed to challenge and develop your child's ability to pay attention, sustain concentration, recall information, solve problems, and creatively respond to novel situations. The cost for these programs ranges from approximately $1,000 to $2,000. Published research studies examining the benefits of these programs have consistently revealed short-term improvement in attention and working memory after 30 to 40 practice sessions (done at least three times per week). In addition, one study demonstrated neurological benefits on a positron emission tomography scan following working memory training. However, a recently published meta-analysis did not find that effects were sustained when treatment was discontinued or transferred to other types of tasks.

The finding that the effects of this type of training decreased when the child stopped training is not surprising to me. Think about the effects of any type of physical exercise. If you went to the YMCA or other fitness center or worked out three or four times a week, your cardiovascular health would improve tremendously. However, if you stopped going to the gym, what would happen? Right: The benefits would wash out. So if you plan on using computerized attention training, think of it as going to a brain gym and find a way to make it part of each day.

What about the lack of transfer to other types of tasks? Again, think about the gym comparison. If you went to a gym and worked on improving lower body strength, would it make you better able to hit a fastball, figure skate, dance, or do other kinds of activities? Probably not. However, my guess is that it would make it more likely that you could learn such skills more easily.

As a result, I encourage parents to explore computerized attention training if they cannot afford or find an EEG biofeedback practitioner. If you can't afford to purchase CogMed or Captain's Log, there is an online training program that is quite affordable and provides similar training. The program is Lumosity (www.lumosity.com), and the cost is approximately $5 to $7 per month. Like other computerized attention and working memory programs, Lumosity is not likely to be a treatment that you can start, stop, and expect sustained gains. However, if you think of it as a portable brain gym that your child can use at least 3 days per week on an ongoing basis, you should anticipate improvement in attention and working memory. Unfortunately, there is little indication that CogMed, Captain's Log, or Lumosity improves symptoms of hyperactivity.

Parents interested in exploring nonmedical strategies for reducing hyperactivity may also find it helpful to consult with an occupational therapist and learn more about movement programs (sometimes called *sensory diets*) that seem to help reduce symptoms of hyperactivity for an hour or two. Just remember, medical and nonmedical treatments for ADHD are not mutually exclusive. Most of my patients use some type of attention training regardless of whether they are being treated with medications for ADHD. We have found that such a combination helps to reduce the amount of medication needed, boosts essential skills, and (in the case of biofeedback) can help to eliminate the need for medication altogether.

Homework

Before you read any further in this book, take a few moments to consider the adequacy of your child's medical treatment for ADHD. If she or he is not taking medication, consider some of the medical options. If you are not comfortable with the use of medication, actively explore one of the psychological treatments that have been found to produce improvements in attention and behavioral control. If your child is taking medication, complete the two rating forms at the end of this lesson and see how your child's treatment is shaping up. If your child is continuing to have significant problems succeeding at home or school, adjustments are needed. Talk about your concerns with your child's doctor, psychologist, counselor, and teacher. See if you can begin to figure out what is going wrong.

In this lesson, I have provided certain guidelines for you to consider. Use them as best as you can, but please do not minimize the importance of effective medical intervention. In my treatment of patients with ADHD, I have learned that when properly administered and monitored, medication can be an essential component in the effective treatment of ADHD. However, when administered without consideration of a child's diet, sleep habits or careful review of other medical problems, the effects can be alarming. Regardless of your degree of comfort about using medication, it is important for you to realize that without addressing the underlying medical factors causing your child's ADHD-like symptoms, even the most judicious use of reminders and consequences is unlikely to be successful.

My bottom-line advice to you is this: Do not accept that your child is untreatable, and do not tolerate the passage of month after month without improvement. People consult with specialists when first-line types of treatment fail. Do not hesitate to do so if the standard type of medical care provided by your child's pediatrician or family practitioner is not working. You are not insulting your doctor by asking for a referral to a consultant for a second opinion. Your child's doctor also wants your child to be well.

Just make sure that the "consultant" is a health care provider who specializes in the treatment of ADHD. Simply because a person is licensed as a psychologist, psychiatrist, or social worker does not mean that he or she is able to provide the range of care needed to treat ADHD. Although you may have some difficulty identifying an ADHD specialist in your region, the clinical psychology, social work, nursing or medical schools at a nearby university or regional teaching hospital can provide you with some potentially useful leads. Although these specialists may be too far from your home for a weekly consultation, remember that they can serve as essential members of your child's treatment team. After a specialist performs an initial evaluation of your child, an ADHD expert can help guide pharmacological, psychological, and educational interventions provided by health care providers in your region. As you will learn in this book, effective treatment of ADHD requires medical interventions, adequate nutrition, school-based accommodation and remediation, systematic use of effective parenting strategies, and training in the development of attention, working memory, problem-solving and social skills.

Medication Tolerance Checklist

CHILD'S NAME: _____ BIRTH DATE: _____

Medications: _____ Dose _____ Times Given: _____

_____ Dose _____ Times Given: _____

_____ Dose _____ Times Given: _____

Name of Prescribing Doctor: _____ Phone: _____

WHICH OF THESE SYMPTOMS DOES YOUR CHILD SHOW? (Check all that apply)

1. _____ Runs about uncontrollably at home in the morning
2. _____ Runs about uncontrollably at home in the afternoon
3. _____ Runs about uncontrollably at home in the evening
4. _____ Appears to be in a fog or dazed in the morning
5. _____ Appears to be in a fog or dazed in the afternoon
6. _____ Appears to be in a fog or dazed in the evening
7. _____ Seems more likely to cry than usual
8. _____ Seems more likely to throw objects, yell at, or hit people than usual
9. _____ Has little or no appetite
10. _____ Is having more difficulty falling asleep at night
11. _____ Has stomach pain or discomfort
12. _____ Has headaches
13. _____ Is drowsy during the day
14. _____ Complains of a dry mouth
15. _____ Is wetting the bed at night
16. _____ Has begun to show a lot of eye blinks, muscle spasms, or shrugs

Other concerns? _____

_____

_____

Please complete this form daily for 5 days. Fax to _____ at the following number _____. Thank you

© Vincent J. Monastra, PhD

Medication Response Chart

PATIENT'S NAME _____ Date: _____

RATER: _____

PLEASE CHECK ONLY WHEN A PROBLEM OCCURS: _____

Time of Day

Behavior	7–9 a.m.	9–11 a.m.	11 a.m.–1 p.m.	1–3 p.m.	3–5 p.m.
Did not listen:					
A little					
A lot					
Interrupts:					
A little					
A lot					
Off task:					
A little					
A lot					
Noisy:					
A little					
A lot					
Moody:					
A little					
A lot					
Hits/Pushes:					
A little					
A lot					
Argues/Defies:					
A little					
A lot					

Please complete this form daily for 5 days. Fax to _____
at the following number: _____. Thank you

© Vincent J. Monastra, PhD

LESSON 4

NUTRITION DOES MATTER

In this lesson, I focus on your child's dietary habits and how they relate to attention, impulsivity, and hyperactivity. Why? Is it because I think that attention-deficit/hyperactivity disorder (ADHD) is caused by inadequate nutrition? No, that's not the reason, although there is evidence that children who have deficiencies of iron, zinc, calcium, magnesium, and vitamin D will show symptoms of inattention, impulsivity, and hyperactivity. Is it because I think that food allergies cause ADHD? Again, the answer is no, although there are well-controlled studies that indicate that symptoms that mimic ADHD can be caused by allergic reactions to foods such as wheat, corn, soy, eggs, milk, nuts, and certain food dyes and additives.

It is important for you to understand how foods contribute to a person's ability to attend, inhibit impulsive behaviors, analyze information, regulate emotional responses, and solve problems. Our selection of foods will determine whether we have the capacity to manufacture the essential neurotransmitters necessary for brain functions. What we eat will determine whether we will have the materials necessary to manufacture the enzymes, cells, and tissues essential for life functions. In addition, should we mistakenly eat foods that cause allergic reactions, our ability to attend, think, and control our emotions will be compromised. Because of this, I routinely request that all of my patients be screened for common food allergies (e.g., corn, wheat, gluten, eggs, dairy, nuts, cocoa, food dyes) before initiating medication for ADHD or making specific dietary recommendations to address nutritional deficiencies.

WHAT KINDS OF NUTRIENTS ARE IMPORTANT FOR THE BRAIN?

This is an important and complex question. I'll try to limit what I review to those types of nutrients that have been investigated in controlled clinical studies of patients who have symptoms of inattention, impulsivity, and hyperactivity. The most critical appear to be the amino acids tyrosine, tryptophan, and phenylalanine (derived from protein-based foods), minerals (e.g., iron, zinc, calcium, magnesium), vitamins (especially vitamin D), and essential fatty acids (EFAs). That is not to say that we do not need to consume foods that contain sodium, potassium, and other vitamins, minerals, and nutrients. It is just important that you realize that deficiencies of certain types of foods can contribute to some of the problems commonly shown by patients with ADHD.

Let's start with proteins. The most common sources of protein are beef, pork, poultry, fish, eggs, beans, nuts, and dairy products. These foods are absorbed by our bodies and used to make neurotransmitters, the chemicals released by our brain cells to communicate with each other so that we can pay attention, learn, solve problems, control our emotional reactions, and do all the other tasks essential for our survival. Without a sufficient amount of protein, it is impossible to pay attention, control our actions, and regulate our moods. Because our bodies immediately begin to make brain-awakening neurotransmitters when you eat protein, a good idea is to start your day with a breakfast that includes milk, cheese, eggs, meat, peanut butter, soy, or a high protein (whey or soy) drink or bar.

What about minerals? We have learned that deficiencies of several minerals can cause symptoms of inattention, impulsivity, and hyperactivity. The minerals that have primarily been studied are iron, zinc, magnesium, and calcium. Let's start with iron because it is a mineral that may be more familiar to you.

Iron can be obtained from a variety of foods. Although spinach has been famous as a good source of iron since the days of the classic cartoon *Popeye*, it is far from the only food that can help us take in our daily requirements of this mineral. Certain cereals (e.g., Cheerios, Frosted Mini-Wheats, Total), meats, vegetables (e.g., peas), and starches (e.g., potatoes) contain iron. Why worry about iron intake? Because iron is directly related to transporting oxygen to the brain. Without oxygen, brain cells are unable to function and will die. Iron is also involved in the production of certain enzymes that are needed to make neurotransmitters like dopamine and serotonin.

Zinc is a mineral that has become a more familiar nutrient over the past few years, particularly for its role in fighting colds, influenza, and infection. Like iron, zinc can be found in cereals like Cheerios, Wheaties, Total, Product 19, and even sugary ones like Cap'n Crunch's Peanut Butter Crunch and Cinnamon Toast Crunch. It can also be found in foods like beef, beans, turkey, chicken, pork, lamb, oysters, and crab. Zinc is an essential ingredient in the development of numerous enzymes, including those that make our neurotransmitters.

Magnesium is a mineral that (like zinc) is involved in hundreds of enzyme activities. In fact, it has been identified in more than 300 enzyme reactions (about half of the known metabolic processes in our bodies). Among the substances that are developed from magnesium are the myelin sheath that surrounds our brain cells (making it possible for neural transmission) and the neurotransmitters involved in attention and concentration. Like other minerals, magnesium is found in meats, nuts, soybeans, and the ever-popular spinach.

Calcium is widely known as a mineral that helps build strong bones, which is true. However, calcium plays an essential role in the release of "brain juice" from one cell to another. When a brain cell is stimulated to fire and release neurotransmitters, tiny calcium channels are opened up at the end of the brain cell. Calcium pours into the cells, tears open tiny sacs of neurotransmitter, and causes the release of neurotransmitters like dopamine and norepinephrine. Without a sufficient amount of calcium, we will have difficulty sustaining attention and controlling our emotional reactions. Most of us know that calcium is readily available in dairy products like milk, cheese, and yogurt and in meats.

Vitamin D is a substance that directly relates to calcium bonding and can have a significant impact on attention. As I mentioned, calcium is essential for releasing the neurotransmitters that help us pay attention. However, vitamin D is the substance that attracts or binds calcium to bones and the endings of brain cells. Without a sufficient amount of vitamin D, the necessary amount of calcium is not available at the endings of brain cells, and our attention, concentration, and mood control suffers. Vitamin D is primarily produced by skin exposure to sunlight. Although a lot of foods containing calcium are enriched with vitamin D (e.g., most dairy products are fortified with vitamin D), people living in regions where the climate reduces the amount of time spent outside with skin exposed to the sunlight are at increased risk for vitamin D deficiencies.

Recently, I gave a workshop to a group of health care providers on Long Island, New York. As I was driving down the road, I noticed a doctor's office with a sign encouraging people to take at least 5,000 IUs of vitamin D per day. That doctor was right on the money. Although some physicians in my region will casually comment that "probably everyone living in the Northeast has a vitamin D deficiency," the fact is that such a deficiency is not something to be ignored. People with such deficiencies are more prone to feel lethargic, inattentive, moody, and seek other types of substances to change this (e.g., alcohol, high-sugar foods, have a "fourth meal" in the evening). Vitamin D supplements are readily available and affordable. For those who have such a deficiency, establishing normal vitamin D levels can have dramatic effects on attention and mood. As a result, screening for these vitamin and mineral deficiencies is a must from my perspective.

EFAs are also important for maintaining attention. They include linoleic acid and alpha-linoleic acids and must be eaten because the body cannot synthesize them. The "n-3" (omega-3) fatty acids are used to build and repair the myelin sheath that surrounds nerve cells. Fish and nuts are an essential source of EFAs. For those allergic to such foods, omega-3 fatty acid supplements are available at most supermarkets, health food stores, and pharmacies.

What Are My Kids Supposed to Eat?

In some ways, you are already an expert on the issue of food and attention. Think about it. What happens if you get up and don't have time to eat breakfast and get to work by eight o'clock? What will you do? Eat a carrot? Nope, not likely. Reach for a cigarette and a cup of coffee? Maybe. Grab a donut? A soda? Again, fairly likely. Why? Because they help you feel more alert . . . for a little while.

When you are feeling sluggish, nothing cures the sense of fatigue and lack of mental energy faster than some carbohydrates (cereal, bagel, or muffin), sugary foods (donut, cookie, or candy bar), some caffeine, or some nicotine. Maybe you didn't realize that sugars are absorbed by brain cells, causing them to become more active. Maybe you didn't know that caffeine and nicotine are central nervous system stimulants that cause an increase in alertness. Even if you didn't know, your body did. Your body also knew that eating a carrot did not immediately increase the activity of brain cells. So there aren't too many of us munching on those in the morning.

However, what most people don't realize is that when they bite into that first donut or munch on a spoonful of cereal, or sip that sugar-laden cup of designer coffee, laced with mocha, drizzled in chocolate, and topped with a mountain of whipped cream, they are setting off a complex series of chemical reactions in the body that will lead them to feel much more drowsy within an hour or so. In our "normal" (unsugared) state, the only region of the body that can use glucose to power cell activity is the brain. But when we eat or drink foods high in glucose, the body senses the arrival of these sugars and starts releasing insulin.

Once insulin is released, it enables every cell in the body to be able to use glucose. Now the brain is competing with gazillions of cells, and glucose availability for brain cells plummets. In addition, the arrival of a high carbohydrate meal at the brain changes which amino acids are permitted to cross the blood–brain barrier. Instead of tyrosine (which we use to make brain-awakening neurotransmitters), the barrier now allows tryptophan (which is used to make brain-calming neurotransmitters) to enter, further sedating your brain. Within an hour or so, you're reaching for another cup of coffee or sugary snack to charge you up again.

Let's shift to lunch. What happens then? Well, for most people, lunch is the first time that they eat any protein. In fact, for many, lunch is the first time that they eat anything other than carbohydrates or sugary sweet drinks. So we head to the various burger worlds, pizza places, or other nearby neighborhood quick eateries to munch. Now I know we want to believe that because we're finally eating all this good stuff (fruits, vegetables, chicken, beef, fish, beans, and breads), after lunch we'll be raring to go. But, as you well know, if we've skipped breakfast, or didn't have a morning meal that included sufficient protein in addition to carbs, we're in a food coma an hour after lunch. Hey, our bodies have to take time to process all that stuff, and it naturally asks for blood to head to the digestive track (which means away from your brain), which is one of the reasons why you're so sluggish. So it's back to caffeine, sugars, and nicotine to survive until we gorge at dinner time and beyond.

Which brings us to the endless feasting that happens after we get home. Many of us will eat while cooking (or waiting for the cooking to be done), have our largest meal of the day at a time our body is preparing to go to sleep, and then wonder why we can't get to sleep until it's midnight (or later). Although we may realize that it's highly unlikely that a body recently filled with sugars (like cereals, chips, dips, crackers, and that "oh so healthy" glass of wine) and caffeine (coffee, colas, and chocolate) will be ready to sleep, these foods taste so good and we deserve to have some fun, right? After we finally get to sleep, we find the alarm going off so early that of course we're not hungry for breakfast. We're mentally and physically fatigued (which certainly doesn't help us concentrate and pay attention). So we gulp down a glass of juice or cup of coffee and the cycle begins again.

The lesson to be learned from all of this is that starting off the day by not eating any protein sets the stage for impaired attention and concentration. For your child to have a chance at being attentive during the morning and throughout the day, nutrition will matter, beginning with breakfast.

So What Do the Experts Recommend?

Most of us are aware that there are governmental agencies that conduct dietary research and are responsible for advising Americans about healthy food choices. Graphic illustrations showing what we should eat have changed over the years. Some of us grew up learning about the Food Pyramid. Now the U.S. Department of Agriculture (USDA) illustrates a healthy meal plan using a plate divided into four sections: grains, vegetables, fruits, and protein. A small circular area on the illustration is labeled *dairy*. The USDA provides detailed recommendations about what a healthy meal plan would look like for children ages 2 through 18. You can find daily food plans, food plan worksheets, and lots of other helpful information online at www.choosemyplate.gov.

Although the emphasis on variety in our children's meal plans is a great idea, kids with ADHD tend to be fairly picky eaters. It is not unusual for children with ADHD to have really strong reactions to the textures of fruits, vegetables, and meats. In addition, because children now are required to wake up and head out to school quite early in the morning, they're often not very hungry in the morning, and if they are taking a stimulant medication, chances are they're not too hungry at lunch. So coming up with a meal plan that includes the foods that are essential for attention can get tricky. That picture of the well-balanced plate may look good on the USDA's Choose-MyPlate website (www.choosemyplate.gov), but making it a reality is going to take some planning, particularly for children who only eat foods that turn into mush once they put them in their mouths.

Let's take a look at what a "mushy-food" kid might have for breakfast. Maybe they get down a breakfast of Cap'n Crunch cereal (.75 cup) and milk (8 oz), have a lunch that includes pizza (two slices) and a soda (12 oz), an after school snack of Doritos (1 oz) and a soda (12 oz), and a dinner that includes spaghetti (1 cup) and meatballs (3.5 oz) with a glass of milk (8 oz). How well would such a meal plan work for a 10-year-old boy weighing 100 pounds? What's your guess? Let's do a simple analysis.

I'll use a standard textbook to determine what is in each of these foods (*Bowes & Church's Food Values of Portions Commonly Used*, Philadelphia: J. B. Lippincott, 1994) and then compare our results with *Dietary Reference Intakes Tables*, authored by the Institute of Medicine of the National Academies (available online at www.iom.edu). If you don't happen to have a personal copy of this book (who does?), you can find the information about the nutritional content of nearly every food at www.nal.usda.gov. There, the USDA publishes the *National Nutrient Database for Standard Reference*. Here is the food comparison:

Daily Food Chart: 10-Year-Old Boy						
Food Content Analysis	**Tryptophan mg**	**Phenylalanine mg**	**Tyrosine mg**	**Iron mg**	**Zinc mg**	**Magnesium mg**
Breakfast:						
Cap'n Crunch	12	76	59	4.81	2.37	10
Milk	113	388	380	0.12	0.95	34
Lunch:						
Pizza (2 slices)	182	732	696	1.16	1.64	32
Soda	0	0	0	0	0	0
Snack:						
Doritos	14	99	82	0.43	0.43	25
Soda	0	0	0	0	0	0
Dinner:						
Spaghetti	85	324	175	1.96	0.74	25
Meatballs	302	929	764	2.10	5.40	20
Milk	113	388	388	0.12	0.95	34
Total Consumed	**821**	**2936**	**2552**	**10.70**	**12.48**	**180**
Advised	**150**	**500**	**500**	**10.00**	**10.00**	**170**

What does this mean? Well, even though our 10-year-old's diet was pretty heavy in terms of calories and fat, his food intake actually exceeds recommended levels for certain amino acids and minerals. While his dietary plan may be far from ideal, it at least contains certain nutrients necessary for brain functioning. The downside is that little was eaten at breakfast. Most was eaten at the end of the day, which really doesn't help with attention and is a great way to put on the pounds.

To help you begin to analyze the adequacy of your child's diet, let's consider the government's recommendations with respect to four basic nutrients that are involved in promoting attention and behavioral control. These nutrients are protein, iron, magnesium, and zinc. The following chart is also derived from the Dietary Reference Intakes developed by the Food and Nutrition Board of the Institute of Medicine (National Academies).

Recommended Daily Dietary Reference Intakes for Protein, Magnesium, Iron, and Zinc					
Group	**Age (years)**	**Protein (g)**	**Magnesium (mg)**	**Iron (mg)**	**Zinc (mg)**
Children	4–8	19	110	4.1	4.0
Males	9–13	34	200	5.9	7.0
Males	14–18	52	340	7.7	8.5
Females	9–13	34	200	5.7	7.0
Females	14–18	46	300	7.9	7.3

Note: Data from *Recommended Dietary Allowances*, by the Food and Nutrition Board, 1989.

As you review this chart, please note that it is intended to provide a general guideline. Specific dietary recommendations are linked to an individual's height and weight. A consultation with a registered dietician is probably wise if you want a thorough analysis of the adequacy of your child's diet. However, if I start examining diet with that type of detail in this book, you're probably going to get lost. Let's try to keep it simple.

How Can I Use These Charts?

A good place to begin is to keep a simple food log for a week. Just so you don't get overwhelmed, start on a weekend. Write down everything your child eats. Try to be as accurate as possible (especially the number of ounces of protein foods). Next, begin to calculate how much protein your child ate. Sometimes the information will be provided on the food wrapper, sometimes it won't. The simplest way to track the amount of protein in foods is the Rule of Sevens. The following amounts of food will provide approximately 7 grams of protein:

- 1 oz of any kind of beef, pork, poultry, fish, or cheese;
- 7 oz of milk (regardless of the fat content);
- one extra large egg; or
- 2 tablespoons of peanut butter.

In addition to these foods, there is a surprisingly high amount of protein found in Greek-style yogurt (15 grams), pizza (typically about 10 grams per slice), or a bagel (about 10 grams). Get your kids involved as detectives "inspecting" the amount of protein in different foods when you go to the grocery store.

How Much Protein Is Enough?

When you look at the Dietary Reference Intakes chart, you'll see total daily amounts (e.g., 19 grams for children ages 4–8; 34 grams for children ages 9–13). Some families find it easy to divide the total amount of recommended protein into thirds and encourage their child to eat approximately one third of the total amount at each meal. In my clinical practice, I typically encourage a higher amount of protein than recommended at breakfast, primarily because patients treated with stimulants will often have little appetite at lunch. The following guide is what we use at my clinic.

This type of guide has been useful for the thousands of patients seen at my clinic. However, if you feel overwhelmed trying to implement this type of program, give yourself a break and obtain an evaluation from a registered dietician. Such a consultation won't cost a lot of money and is likely to provide you with useful information, as well

Recommended Intakes of Protein for Breakfast and Lunch		
Age group	Gender	Protein (g): Breakfast/lunch
4–8	Male or female	10 grams/10 grams
9–13	Male or female	20 grams/20 grams
14+	Male	25 grams/25 grams
14+	Female	20 grams/20 grams

as with some strategies for improving your child's diet. If the goal is to improve your child's attention and impulse control, you need to make sure they are eating the kinds of foods that will help them develop these skills. No amount of medication, parenting, school intervention, or counseling will correct an attention problem that is caused by nutritional deficiency.

To set the stage for improved protein intake at breakfast, it is important for parents to begin to establish a bedtime routine that will provide a sufficient amount of sleep for their child. Exhausted, tired, sleep-deprived children have little appetite in the morning. If their breakfast meal consists of stimulant medication and water, you are headed for trouble. To enhance attention and reduce risk for adverse medication reactions because of sleep deficits and dietary insufficiency, I recommend that children in the primary grades attain at least 10 hours of sleep per night, and adolescents attain at least 8 hours of sleep per night. Children and adolescents getting less than 7 hours of sleep per night are likely to have attention and mood problems that have more to do with sleep deficits and less to do with ADHD than you'd think.

From my perspective, sleep deficits are the joker in the deck when it comes to treating ADHD. Unless sleep problems are addressed, it is difficult to treat attention problems through medication. If your child has a hard time settling down, consider eliminating exposure to any type of video screens (and that includes the vast array of smartphones) for at least 1 hour before bedtime. A high carbohydrate snack before bed (e.g., ice cream, milk and cereal, cheese and crackers) can also help. If neither of these approaches work (and your child is eating sufficient protein at breakfast) a brief trial of a melatonin supplement (e.g., 1–3 mg administered 1.5–2.0 hours before bedtime) can help. If none of these strategies is sufficient to treat sleep deficits, then a trial of an antihypertensive medication like clonidine or guanfacine in the evening may be beneficial until healthy sleep habits have been established.

What If My Kid Won't Eat Anything Worthwhile?

This is probably the most common complaint I hear from the parents of my patients. I wish I could tell you that if you just ignored the issue, it would go away. It doesn't. Among the thousands of kids I have treated, I have rarely met a child who ate a sufficient amount of protein at breakfast and lunch. A lot of my patients are pretty much zombies in the morning and get so distracted by the activity in the cafeteria that they forget to eat lunch. In addition, the appetite of kids who are being treated with a stimulant will be suppressed because of medication effects.

So to get things moving in the right direction, you will need to make a decision. If you accept the scientific evidence that indicates the brain actually needs foods that provide essential amino acids, vitamins, and minerals, then you will need to make eating a nutritious breakfast and lunch one of the lessons to be learned in life. While your child will need to be involved in choosing protein-rich foods that will provide a variety of amino acids, vitamins, and minerals, you will need to establish the ground rules. In some ways, family rules about nutrition are going to sound similar to those you probably have for bathing, brushing teeth, and bedtime.

Just as brushing teeth, taking a shower, and getting enough sleep are essential, so is eating a nutritious breakfast and lunch. As with these other areas, choosing not to follow Mom's and Dad's rules is not OK. Your child will need to learn that the use of electronic entertainment devices (e.g., television, computer, video games, smartphones) and permission to engage in desirable activities (e.g., playing outside, visiting friends, going to baseball or soccer practice, attending dance class) are linked to dietary habits. I have often said to kids, "If your brain is running on empty because you haven't fed it enough protein, then you really should be resting." A father of one of my patients put it even better. He told his son, "If you're not putting fuel for your brain into your body, then I'm not putting fuel in the car to drive you to practice." He was serious. It worked.

Protein-Rich Foods That Kids With ADHD Might Eat in the Morning

The heart of the solution to the breakfast war centers on two simple truths: First, dietary protein at breakfast and lunch is important for attention. There's no getting around this, and a great dinner doesn't make up for a lousy breakfast. Second, kids with ADHD will need to have easily digestible and desirable foods available to them for their morning meal. Fighting endlessly to get your child to eat that last morsel of the one egg he hates will just wear you out and make the cereal aisle look like an oasis. The following list comes from my patients. You might find some foods that will appeal to even the pickiest kid. One truism about kids with ADHD: Nothing works forever. My patients may love a particular food for months and then tire of it. I hope this list will give you some workable options for those moments.

MEATS. Sausage links, sausage biscuits, bacon, Slim Jim beef jerky and beef sticks, and chicken nuggets are OK with many of my kids. Nontraditional breakfast foods such as hot dogs, a burger, or a burrito can work as well. Some of my patients love beef, chicken, or pork lo mein. In a rush, a slice of deli ham, turkey, or chicken can work. Remember, each ounce of meat provides about 7 grams of protein.

EGGS. A couple of eggs (cooked any way that will go down) are a good way to get started. You can cut the white portion of a hard-boiled egg down into soft little protein chunks. One of my kids liked it mixed with applesauce (believe it or not). An extra-large egg white provides about 7 grams of protein.

DAIRY. An 8-oz glass of milk beats walking out the door with nothing in the stomach (it gives your child 8 grams of protein). Cheese sticks go down pretty well, and every ounce of cheese provides about 7 grams. Yogurt is also easily tolerated and you can boost the protein level by mixing in some whey-based protein powder or a little dry milk. Cheese sandwiches (grilled or not) may also be a winner. I often gross out my patients with my morning favorite: cold lasagna (spaghetti and meatballs and scrambled eggs with hot dog slices are tied for second). Pizza (in all varieties) can work as well. An almost universally accepted morning meal is a scoop of ice cream (any kind) mixed with a capful of an unflavored whey powder. This turns the ice cream into a soft serve and is really, really good. Most protein powders provide at least 15 grams of protein.

NUTS. Peanut butter on toast, crackers, a bagel, or a muffin isn't too tough a sell. Kids can smear on all the jelly or marshmallow fluff they want. Some kids will prefer just munching on nuts. You'd be surprised how few nuts make up a serving (about 15 nuts or 2 tablespoons of peanut butter provide about 7 grams of protein). A lot of kids also like adding peanut butter to a 6- to 8-oz chocolate milk shake (with a little protein powder added by Mom or Dad).

Soy. There are a number of soy protein powders available for mixing in drinks and using in recipes. Very few of my patients can tolerate a drink made from those bodybuilding-type powders (too chalky—the kids feel like they are gagging). The same is true for most protein bars (too dense for my patients). However, many of my patients love Special K's Protein Bars (I eat them like candy), and Cliff Bars are generally well liked. Snicker's Marathon Bar is also pretty tasty. If your child is lactose intolerant and soy is one of the ways you'd like to go, think baking. Many of my patients have parents who will creatively combine soy powder with flour, sugar, baking powder and other ingredients to make high-protein chocolate chip cookies, muffins, brownies, and a variety of fruit breads (apple, banana). This is one of the easiest ways to get 10 to 20 grams of protein into your child. These treats are easily transportable to school for lunch and snack. Just make sure that your soy powder can be used in cooking.

Meals for Kids With Absolutely No Appetite

You've just read this list and said to yourself "None of these will work!" I know; it can happen. Here are two nearly foolproof ideas. First, because some of my patients simply feel ill at the thought of food in the morning, I have searched for light, easily digestible drinks. There are two winners, according to my patients. Gatorade's G-3 and Ensure Light are fruit-based liquids that are not heavy. They have around

15 grams of protein per serving. I've found that teenage boys and girls are not at all embarrassed to carry around a G-3 drink at school and sip through the day. When you combine a light, fruit drink with a Special K Protein Bar or a Cliff Bar, you've got a 25-gram protein meal that's basically a protein candy bar and a fruit drink. Definitely worth considering for breakfast and/or lunch for kids with no appetite.

My favorite recipe for kids combines several of the protein sources and was created by one of my patients who had no appetite. I call it Sean's Breakfast Surprise. It is created from the following ingredients: chocolate pudding, soy protein powder, Cool Whip or other imitation whipped cream, and crushed Oreo cookies. He makes a week's worth of these on Sunday night and freezes them. In the morning, he has one, washes it down with a glass of milk, and is set. This breakfast has a high protein content and great staying power. I mention this one to you as well so that you begin to get the idea that I'm hoping that breakfast can be a bit more creative than bacon and eggs. I'm not rooting for this to be a battle. I hope that as you review the food ideas for breakfast, you and your child will hit on some that will work.

Isn't It a Bad Idea to Make an Issue Out of Eating?

No! Teaching your children about healthy choices is one of a parent's primary roles in life. When parents tell me they are worried that their child will develop an eating disorder because they are insisting on a breakfast meal that includes protein, I usually ask them if they believe their child will become obsessive–compulsive if they make sure the child takes a bath, brushes his or her teeth, or changes into clean clothes. Obviously, there are extreme and abusive methods for teaching lessons about nutrition or cleanliness. I'm not advocating that you make mealtimes anxiety-provoking experiences. I'm simply talking about using common reinforcement strategies to encourage your child to learn an important lesson: Nutrition does count.

What About Allergies?

A review of the scientific literature reveals that well-controlled studies have reported that certain children are sensitive (and become inattentive or hyperactive) when exposed to certain food dyes and preservatives. Other studies indicate that some children demonstrate symptoms of ADHD after ingesting certain foods (e.g., corn, wheat), which is why we routinely request blood screening for common food allergies before initiating treatment for ADHD. If you notice that your child's attention or behavior worsens after eating a specific food, a consultation with an allergist (particularly one familiar with behavioral issues) may be beneficial. The Feingold Association (www.feingold.org) is another excellent source of information on this topic.

HOMEWORK

Take a look at the protein content contained in your child's breakfast. Compare it with the recommended amount. Then have a conversation with your child about the need to have the recommended amount for breakfast each day. Talk with your child about the kinds of foods that can provide the necessary protein. Let him or her help you to decide on the foods that will be available at breakfast. However, let your child know that the new family rule is that he or she needs to eat a nutritious breakfast to have the energy (and your permission) to engage in certain activities. Although I'll be talking about the whole issue of motivating kids with ADHD in later lessons, see how you do in motivating your child to improve his or her diet. Remember, to learn a new skill, children not only need to be shown (or told) the lesson, they also need a reason to try the new skill. That's where motivation comes in.

LESSON 5

STUDENTS WITH ADHD ARE ENTITLED TO HELP AT SCHOOL

One of the most frustrating experiences parents face is the ongoing problem of trying to help children with ADHD succeed in school. Few children diagnosed with ADHD are able to succeed in school without some type of support. For some children, the support is provided by a parent who stays on top of the child from the minute the kid hits the door after school until the time she or he goes to sleep. These parents repeatedly remind the child about homework assignments and plead, argue, fight, punish, praise, and exhaust themselves in an effort to make sure that homework is completed.

For other children, support comes from an understanding teacher who recognizes that the student has problems listening to instructions, remembering assignments, concentrating while reading and writing, organizing books and homework, and keeping up with long-term projects. These teachers independently make accommodations, kindly developing ways for the student with ADHD to be successful without humiliating or criticizing the child. Such educators have recognized that ADHD is a disabling medical condition, just like hearing or visual loss. They have incorporated the knowledge that led our government to determine that ADHD was a health impairment and treat children who have ADHD with the same kind of respect and compassion that would be given to a child who has difficulty in school because of a hearing or visual problem. These teachers are a blessing for kids with ADHD because they recognize that repeated school failure does not breed success. They well know that it leads a child to stop trying and perhaps even drop out of school.

However, despite two federal laws (Individuals With Disabilities Education Act [IDEA]: 2004; and Section 504 of the Rehabilitation Act of 1973) that specify that children with ADHD are entitled to academic support and accommodation, many children with this disorder do not receive any type of support. As an example of how this typically happens, I'll use a patient of mine whom I'll call Mike. His story is similar to those I have heard of thousands of teens with ADHD.

As you read Mike's story, you might consider it to be a bit extreme. However, his experience is far more representative of what occurs in clinical practice than you would think. It is the story of a child described as hyperactive and impulsive who was never diagnosed with ADHD. A similar tale could be told of the child (often a girl) described as inattentive who daydreamed her way through the primary and secondary grades, never realizing her intelligence and never experiencing the satisfaction that comes with school success because she, too, was never diagnosed with ADHD.

Mike came with his parents to my clinic during the 10th grade. He was failing math, science, social studies, Spanish, and English. He did not complete assignments, did not study for tests, and routinely cut classes. Because of his illegal absences from class, he would routinely be placed in in-school suspension, reporting to a specific room where he was to remain all day. However, he would feel restless being cooped up in such a place and would avoid going there. As a result, further disciplinary action would occur, typically out-of-school suspension, which is like getting a week of school vacation as a reward for misbehavior. In addition to being ineffective (because it rewards misbehavior), such a disciplinary action is potentially dangerous for a teenager whose parent or guardian can't be home during the day and can't afford other supervision.

Of course, Mike's school problems were not limited to merely cutting classes and getting bad grades. He made jokes and talked in class, interrupting the teacher and class activities. But none of this is what brought Mike to my clinic. What did? His temper.

In many schools across the country, the junior and senior high school years are times when a kid has to handle a lot of "meanness." Most of us don't have to deal with someone teasing or threatening us at work on a day-to-day basis, because our country has laws against those kinds of behaviors in the workplace. However, for quite some time, our children did not have that same degree of protection. Now the federal government has begun to take a stand against those types of behaviors in schools. Although there is no specific federal law that specifically prohibits bullying, the U.S. Department of Education and the U.S. Department of Justice now enforce federal civil rights laws (e.g., Title IV and Title VI of the Civil Rights Act of 1964) and the Americans With Disabilities Act when discriminatory harassment occurs in schools.

As a result, each school district in our country is required to develop policies to protect every student from the actions of peers that create a persistently hostile environment that is sufficiently serious to interfere with a student's ability to participate in the programs offered by a school. In my home state (New York), the Dignity for All Students Act serves as the foundation for school policy relating to bullying. Your home state has similar laws protecting your child as well. The goals of all of these legislative initiatives are to create school environments free of discrimination and harassment and to require school districts to develop antibullying programs and policies. If your child is the target of bullying, you do not have to simply hope and wait for things to change. Your district in all likelihood has a specific policy and procedure for filing reports. You need to find out the procedure and initiate the steps to protect your child, immediately.

Unfortunately, this type of process wasn't in place when Mike was in school. Like many kids in Grades 7 through 12 (and in the earlier grades as well), Mike faced daily mocking comments, social isolation, and verbal and physical threats. And he didn't know how to handle them. If you're a kid with ADHD (meaning you have impulse control problems and difficulty finding the words that you need to solve problems), you are going to have a hard time figuring out what to do when you are teased and threatened. It is also likely that you will be subjected to some type of disciplinary action because of impaired impulse control. That's what happened to Mike.

In Mike's case, someone made one too many wisecracks in a classroom. Mike threw some tables and chairs and was headed for the kid, threatening to kill him. Not a smart thing to do. The net result: Mike was expelled from school, pending consultation with a doctor like me. His parents and teachers were unsure what was wrong. Some thought he was emotionally disturbed and needed to be placed in a hospital for intensive treatment. Some thought he was on drugs. Others felt he was depressed. The ever-popular oppositional-defiant disorder was suggested as an explanation for his academic and social problems. Perhaps it was his parents' fault for being too easy on Mike. Not a single teacher suggested ADHD. If they had taken a look at his academic history, all of them would have.

Mike's kindergarten teacher initially noted that he was a kid who had difficulty remaining seated, particularly during group activities. He would interrupt instruction, provide answers before questions were completed, and intrude on others as they worked. He seemed to have a hard time listening and needed to be busy. She recognized his intelligence and considered him to be an enthusiastic student who needed to slow down a bit.

During the primary grades, Mike continued to display difficulties remaining on task during group instruction. He was fidgety in his seat and had to be reminded to be quiet during class. His desk was a mess, and he had a hard time finding materials. He forgot papers that needed to get to his parents and lost homework that needed to be returned to his teachers. However, the results of standardized tests of academic skills indicated that he was a bright child with no evidence of a learning disorder. His teachers thought so too, although his work was sloppy, and his handwriting was hard to decipher. During these years, he was considered to be an intelligent child who needed to concentrate and work harder. His parents were given the impression that Mike could do better if he tried. Mike began to be punished at home for failing to do his best, but the punishment did little to change his behavior or performance at school.

By the time Mike hit the third and fourth grades, teachers were no longer making positive comments on his report cards. Rather, he would learn that his report card marks were lowered by his failure to complete assignments. He was told that he needed to work harder. His report cards would include long checklists of skills needing improvement (e.g., does not listen, does not complete work assigned in class, lacks self-control). His work continued to be sloppy, and his lack of motivation was cause for concern.

During this time, daily notes were exchanged between parents and teachers about assignments, and each day was a battle between Mike and his parents. To get Mike to complete his work, one of his parents would have to sit with him. The parent would need to prompt Mike repeatedly to do his work. However, Mike would complain that he didn't know what to do or how to find the answers to the questions in English, science, or social studies. Getting some kind of answer on paper was even more of a problem. Mike would drive his parents crazy with his inability to recognize an answer, even when they pointed out the information in his book. His one-to-three-word answers came after hours of work. Even more frustrating, after all the time and effort expended by his parents, Mike often lost his homework. In addition, his lack of knowledge of basic facts made completing his math homework an exercise in creative guessing.

During junior high, the bottom fell out. He had a different teacher for each subject. His lack of interest in schoolwork, his failure to complete assignments, and his low test scores resulted in failing grades. His classroom interruptions were no longer considered evidence of intelligence and enthusiasm. They simply resulted in disciplinary actions. Progress notes from teachers indicated that he needed to pay attention, study harder, and complete his work. "Junior high is the time when kids need to take responsibility for their actions," they'd say. If Mike did not make the effort, then he would fail and attend summer school. Maybe failure and spending part of his summer vacation in school would turn the tide. Of course, it didn't.

When you review these teacher comments, nearly every one of Mike's teachers from kindergarten on up noticed that this child had difficulty attending to instruction, concentrating on school tasks, completing work, organizing his materials, and controlling impulsive behavior. Yet he was never identified as a student with ADHD. One question screams for an answer: How did Mike's ADHD go undiagnosed for so long?

Although there are many ways this question could be answered, I think it boils down to the lack of what doctors call a *diagnostic formulation*. Let me tell you what a diagnostic formulation is. It's a fancy way to answer the question "Why is this person having these problems?" In Mike's case, no qualified health care professional was asked to conduct a thorough evaluation to determine the causes of his ADHD symptoms until he was 16 years old. Without such an evaluation and diagnostic formulation, children with any kind of medical problem will continue to struggle with their symptoms.

That shouldn't surprise anyone, whether we are talking about visual or hearing impairments, respiratory or heart problems, or attention and impulse control disorders.

When we are talking about children who show symptoms of inattention, hyperactivity, and impulsivity, parents and teachers try to determine why the child is not succeeding. This is understandable. It certainly makes sense that for a 6-month period, teachers and parents explore issues such as academic skill development, maturity, and motivation as they attempt to improve a child's attention, concentration, and behavioral control. However, if ADHD symptoms have persisted in a child who is age 4 years or older for longer than 6 months despite the best effort of parents and teachers, and it is the opinion of the teacher that the child's inattention or lack of behavioral control is atypical for her or his age and is interfering with learning or educational performance, it is time to seek an evaluation by a qualified health care specialist.

The reasons for evaluation by a psychologist, clinical social worker, or physician (usually a pediatrician, family practitioner, or psychiatrist) go back to the idea of a diagnostic formulation. Teachers can evaluate a child's abilities in reading, mathematics, and written expression, helping to identify children who are not paying attention because of learning disabilities. They can also provide valuable information regarding a child's behavior and functioning in the class. By doing so, they can assist a doctor in determining the presence of ADHD symptoms in the classroom. However, as I reviewed in previous lessons, symptoms of inattention, hyperactivity, and impulsivity can be caused by a variety of medical conditions, including ADHD. Teachers are not certified to diagnose the reasons a child is displaying symptoms of inattention, impulsivity or hyperactivity; doctors are. It simply is not appropriate for teachers to be placed (or to place themselves) in a position to diagnose ADHD. They do not have the training, the expertise, or the professional license to do so.

HOW CAN I GET MY KID HELP IN SCHOOL?

After your child is diagnosed with ADHD by a qualified health care professional, he or she can receive assistance at school for problems with attention and behavioral control. It is important for you to realize that the federal government considers ADHD to be a health condition that can limit alertness for academic tasks and adversely affect educational performance (IDEA PL 108-446) as well as a medical-psychiatric condition that can impair learning, a significant life function (Section 504 of the Rehabilitation Act of 1973). Because of the preponderance of scientific evidence that ADHD is "real," federal laws require school districts to systematically evaluate children who have been diagnosed with ADHD to determine the ways their health problems are impairing learning or adversely affecting educational performance. Before I get into specific ways to help your child, I'd like to briefly summarize these laws so you better understand the educational rights of children with ADHD.

IDEA

This federal law was initially developed in 1990 so children with disabilities could participate in an educational program that will promote their success. Over the years, this law has been revised several times. The most recent revision of IDEA in 2004 continues to provide funds for school districts to offer specialized educational services for children who have learning disabilities, serious emotional problems, mental retardation, traumatic brain injury, vision or hearing impairment, physical disabilities, or other health problems like ADHD. For a child with ADHD to qualify for supportive services under IDEA, two important conditions must be met. First, the child must be diagnosed with ADHD by a person qualified to do so (e.g., a licensed psychologist, social worker, physician). Second, the ADHD symptoms must be shown to limit alertness to academic tasks and adversely affect educational performance. This is where all those teacher comments on report cards, assignments workbooks, and failure notices can be used to help qualify your child for assistance.

The revision of the IDEA that defined ADHD as a health impairment represented a significant step forward in efforts to help students with ADHD. Before the 1998 revision, some school districts insisted that the child had to be diagnosed with a specific learning disability to receive services. As a result, when parents requested an evaluation for their child with ADHD, tests of intelligence and academic skills were performed. If the results of the testing did not reveal a disability of reading, mathematics, or writing skills, no services were provided. Rarely did school districts inform parents that their children qualified for accommodation under another federal law (the Rehabilitation Act of 1973, Section, 504). As a result, neither remediation nor accommodation was provided to these children.

The revised IDEA clearly states that ADHD is a health impairment and that children do not need to show evidence of a learning disability on standardized tests to qualify for services. Rather, just as with children who are deaf or blind, children with ADHD are entitled to a *functional assessment*. School districts are required to thoroughly assess how a child's attention problems or hyperactivity-impulsivity are interfering with educational performance and to develop an educational plan of instruction and accommodation that is sufficient for the child to succeed in school. Let's take a minute to think through this by comparing a patient with ADHD and one who is not succeeding because of a hearing loss.

Picture yourself as the parent of a child whose hearing is significantly impaired. You know that your child has difficulty listening and cannot follow verbal instructions, but sometimes he seems as though he understands what you're talking about. Let's pretend that this child somehow ends up in school and no one knows that she or he had a hearing loss. The child might move about the class, unaware that the teacher is asking him or her to sit down. The child would not hear the teacher's instructions and would not remember. This forgetfulness would lead to reprimands (and disciplinary action) from the teacher, failure to complete assignments, and poor marks on report cards. If you and the teacher followed my 6-month rule, your child would be evaluated by a physician or other specialist, and the hearing loss would be identified. This information would be shared with your child's school district and an Individualized Education Plan (IEP) would be developed.

After the plan was developed and implemented in the classroom, life would greatly change for the better. No longer would you and the teacher discuss whether the child's apparent inattention, poor academic performance, or wandering in class was because of a lack of motivation, immaturity, or poor parenting. Instead, you and the teacher would accept the diagnostic formulation of a hearing loss. Your child would no longer be required to "listen" to get instructions. The child would not be told that third-graders should be able to remember what their teachers say and to try harder. Assistive technology (e.g., amplification of the teacher's voice, use of hearing aids) might be used. Instructions given verbally could also be provided in a written form. Testing modifications (e.g., use of written tests only) might also be provided. In short, any and all reasonable accommodations and interventions would be provided so that your child's hearing loss would not interfere with the performance of essential educational tasks.

Now let's imagine your child has problems in attending that are not due to a hearing loss. Let's say you consulted with a doctor and learned that the child's inattention was caused by a different type of health impairment, ADHD. Now what? Well, just as with a hearing loss, the school district would need to be informed of the diagnosis. And, just as with a hearing loss, the school district would need to conduct a thorough evaluation of the ways ADHD was affecting the child's educational performance and provide assistance.

This means that parents of children with ADHD no longer need to accept that a school will not provide assistance because the test results showed that their child did not have a learning disability. All too often, parents have accepted that their child simply needed to try harder to control him- or herself and try to pay attention. From my perspective (and that of the federal government), that would be the same as telling a child with hearing impairment that he needs to try to listen better or a child with a visual impairment that she needs to try to see better. Kids with hearing or visual impairments are entitled to better treatment . . . so are kids with ADHD!

What Kind of Help Is Available for Children With ADHD?

A lot. I'll give you a brief overview now and get specific later in this lesson. Children with ADHD are likely to have specific disabilities in reading, mathematics, and written expression. Hence, part of their educational program will involve efforts to improve those skills. They may participate in remedial reading, writing, or mathematics through Academic Intervention Services at their school or may receive more individualized instruction in those skills from special education teachers. Many schools have adopted a Response to Intervention (RTI) model, which creates a three-tiered approach that provides a more systematic strategy for helping children who are having difficulty learning, regardless of whether or not they have a specific learning disability or health impairment.

The emphasis of the RTI model is to encourage school districts to use empirically based remediation strategies in class instruction for all students (Tier 1), in small group instruction (Tier 2), or in more individualized instruction (Tier 3) to maximize learning. However, it is important for parents to realize that RTI is a regular education intervention. It is not intended to replace the IDEA as the foundation of services for students with qualifying conditions (including ADHD). The IDEA requires comprehensive individual education plans that target all areas of functional impairment related to ADHD in a specific child.

For example, children with ADHD who also display significant problems on tests of reading skills won't succeed if they are given one period of remedial reading per day and are then sent home to read their seventh-grade social studies book, search for the answers to the questions listed in the back of their chapter, and write down the answers for the 20 homework questions. If their reading ability is impaired, then their educational plan must include not only remediation, but also accommodations (or adjustments). The same holds true if the disability is in the area of mathematics or written expression. A listing of many of these accommodations is provided at the end of this lesson.

Whereas many children with ADHD have specific learning disabilities, others do not. These children have academic performance problems that are not directly related to their ability to read, write, or answer math problems per se. Rather, these children have difficulties attending to instruction, concentrating while reading, and remembering and organizing information while writing. In addition, children with ADHD are easily distracted by other children and activities in and around the classroom. They drift off and do not hear the teacher's instructions. They find it difficult to remain in their seats. They interrupt the teacher and other students. They are unable to concentrate or complete seat work like other children and end up losing recess time or have to stay after school to complete their work. They find that they cannot write as quickly and neatly as others and end up having to redo their work. They struggle to succeed in so many ways—and there are so many ways that you and their school can help.

Both remediation and accommodation are the keys to succeeding in school. A teacher has every right to decide that she or he will try to help students learn essential facts in social studies by asking them to find the answers to a list of questions. However, if a child has ADHD, this instructional method will need to be modified to accommodate the child's medical abilities and limitations. Just as a teacher would not be likely to ask a student with a hearing impairment to take notes in class and study them for a test, a teacher of a student with ADHD is required to make similar accommodations.

When I speak with parents and teachers about such accommodations, there is often a sense of resistance. Sometimes, the hesitancy is framed as "we can't continue to baby this student." Sometimes, it is expressed as "students in the fifth grade are required to . . . " Sometimes, it is stated as "the student has to learn how to do this sooner or later. They won't give her this type of help in college." Each of these statements reflects a lack of recognition of ADHD as a type of health impairment.

Would you say to a deaf child with hearing impairment, "Look, sooner or later you're going to have to hear. So we are not going to give you class notes in written form anymore"? Would you say to a visually impaired child, "Look, you have got to work harder at reading. You're not going to be able to get audio books forever"? Of course not.

When this same type of reasoning is applied to kids with ADHD, there seems to be an emotional reaction. Sort of like, "Yes, I recognize that the student has ADHD, but he needs to learn how to take his own notes in class." My response is that it would be great if the student can learn how to take notes in class. The student should be taught how to do that. However, until the student demonstrates sufficient ability in that area, the child is entitled to receive assistance and accommodations. To say that a 15-year-old student with ADHD should be able to take notes, organize materials, prepare study guides, study for exams, comprehend literature, and write coherent essays is the equivalent of saying that a visually impaired student should be able to see by the age of 15 years.

ADHD is a health impairment that has been shown to endure into adulthood. Although individuals with ADHD can learn essential academic skills, they do not develop them at the same rate as their peers, nor do they always develop these skills.

As a result, accommodation and remediation efforts are available to these students through college and in work settings. Study guides, note takers, tutors, audio books, the use of computerized systems that can present, highlight, and read any printed material to your child (e.g., Kurzweil Text Reading Software, Read & Write: Gold Edition), use of web-based informational sites, electronic versions of books to simplify information searchers, the use of word-processing software and voice-recognition technology to facilitate writing (e.g., Via Voice or Dragon's Naturally Speaking), the availability of portable word-processing equipment in the classroom (e.g., DreamWriter, AlphaSmart, or laptop computers), testing modifications, and homework accommodations are all permissible through the college and postgraduate level in the United States.

What is the reason for all this help? The IDEA, which specifies that individuals with handicapping conditions cannot be subjected to discrimination. ADHD is considered to be among the qualifying conditions under this law. Individuals who are unable to read because of dyslexia are entitled to be educated in a manner that accommodates (and if possible, remediates) the disability. However, if such individuals are never able to read, they should not be prevented from becoming a doctor, lawyer, or any other chosen career simply because their educational setting refuses to provide accommodations for their instructional limitations. To do so is in violation of federal law. To learn more about IDEA 2004, visit the IDEA website (http://www.ed.gov/policy/speced/guid/idea/idea2004.html).

How Can I Apply This to My Child?

To begin the process of obtaining help for your child, she or he needs to have been diagnosed with ADHD by a qualified health care professional (typically a physician or a licensed psychologist or clinical social worker). After your child is diagnosed with ADHD, you'll need to make a written request for an evaluation by your school district's Committee on Special Education (CSE). The letter should be addressed to the chairperson of the CSE. This person is sometimes referred to as the *director of special education services* or the *director of student services*. Although districts may differ regarding the title given to the person responsible for organizing the evaluation, every school district that receives federal or state funds for education must have such a committee and a person responsible for conducting meetings to develop a plan of academic remediation, support, and accommodation (as needed). An example of such a letter is provided here.

I strongly recommend that this type of letter be sent by certified mail to the chairperson of the CSE or the director of special education services. This individual is required by law to proceed with an evaluation once a written referral is made and documentation of the diagnosis of ADHD is provided. I have seen years wasted by parents talking with their child's teachers, guidance counselors, or principal about getting services for their child. Although I am in support of collaboration between parents, teachers, principals, counselors, and the school psychologist during the first 6 months that symptoms of ADHD become cause for concern, I do not believe that the best interest of the child is served by delaying referral to the CSE if problems at school persist beyond that time frame.

It has been alarming to me how many children display significant attention and behavioral control in kindergarten yet somehow make it to middle school without ever being referred to the CSE.

Sample Letter to the Committee on Special Education (CSE)

Date:

To: Chairperson of the CSE

From: Mr. and Mrs. B.

Re: Timothy B.

Dear _____

My child, Timothy B., was recently evaluated by Dr. Monastra, a licensed psychologist. Based on an extensive review of medical, developmental, academic, and social histories; evaluation of behavioral ratings provided by us and Timothy's teachers; and psychological assessment of Timothy's attention, Dr. Monastra diagnosed our child with attention-deficit/ hyperactivity disorder (ADHD). A copy of Dr. Monastra's report is included with this letter in support of the diagnosis.

As required by federal and state law, we are requesting an evaluation by our school district's Committee on Special Education Services. It is our understanding that because our child has been diagnosed with ADHD, testing for specific learning disabilities and a functional assessment to determine the ways that our son's ADHD is interfering with school performance are required. We are requesting that both be conducted so that an Individualized Education Plan (IEP) or a 504 Accommodation Plan can be developed, depending on my child's needs. A copy of a Functional Assessment Checklist for Teachers (FACT) is included to aid in the evaluation process.

Thank you for your prompt attention to this request.

Sincerely,

Mr. and Mrs. B.

© Vincent J. Monastra, PhD

Yet if parents do not obtain a thorough evaluation by a health care provider licensed to make a diagnosis of ADHD, this is exactly what happens far too often. It is important for you to realize that once your child has been diagnosed with ADHD, a health care provider has determined that he or she has a qualifying health condition. The function of the CSE is not to validate this diagnosis. Rather, its responsibility is to assess the kinds of impairments of learning and educational performance that are present and to develop an IEP or 504 Accommodation Plan. Your certified letter ensures that there is no misunderstanding about the timing and nature of the parents' request and the school's legal requirements.

After you have mailed the letter to the school district, you will be contacted and asked to sign a form that permits evaluation by the CSE. You are also likely to be asked to provide the district with information about your child's medical, developmental, and social histories. This information may be obtained through an interview or by asking you to complete detailed questionnaires.

The evaluation at school will often include individual testing of your child's intelligence, as well as her or his abilities in the areas of reading decoding, reading comprehension, computation, mathematical reasoning, listening comprehension, and written expression. This testing is typically performed by a school psychologist or a special education teacher. In addition, the school psychologist will often conduct a classroom observation, and questionnaires evaluating your child's behavior in the classroom will be completed by his or her teacher(s). Finally, I request that teachers complete a functional Assessment Checklist for Teachers (a copy is provided later in this lesson) so that each area of functional impairment can be identified and subsequently addressed in the child's educational plan.

One of the most important services a psychologist (or other expert) can provide is attendance at the CSE meeting. Because the psychologist (or other expert) that you bring to the meeting should be knowledgeable about ADHD and educational law, he or she can assist the committee in developing a comprehensive plan that will promote your child's academic success. This expert can also provide you with some much-needed support during a meeting that is often overwhelming and intimidating to parents. However, as you participate in the CSE meeting, it is essential to keep in mind that the diagnosis of ADHD qualifies your child for assistance. Your child's entitlement to accommodation or assistance is not a matter for debate. What is up for discussion are the types of accommodations or assistance that will be needed to promote your child's success.

During the meeting, each member of the committee will present test results and observations (as will you and any consultants that accompany you). If there is sufficient evidence that your child's health impairment is affecting his or her alertness in school (e.g., doesn't complete assignments in class, is distracted, does not take accurate class notes, fails to remember books, forgets homework, doesn't follow directions, takes hours to complete assignments that other kids finish in 15 minutes, is unable to develop and use study guides) and that report card grades or other indicators of educational performance are adversely affected by this lack of alertness, then your child's ADHD is a health impairment that meets IDEA requirements. The next step is for the committee to develop a plan of remediation, support, and accommodation, depending on the severity of the functional impairments. The district is required to develop a program that addresses each of the child's functional impairments. The CSE will develop a plan that is the least restrictive option to ensure that the child can benefit from as many of the programs available in the general education setting as possible before providing special education services. However, if the program that is developed is not promoting your child's success, you can request a meeting to revise the IEP or 504 Plan at any time by writing to the CSE chairperson.

To help school districts evaluate the type and severity of a student's functional problems, I developed (and copyrighted) the Functional Assessment Checklist for Teachers (FACT). A copy of the FACT is provided in this lesson for your use. The purpose of the form is to help teachers and the CSE evaluate functional impairments in a systematic manner so that a comprehensive program can be developed for your child. This form should be distributed to all of your child's teachers and the results shared with your child's psychologist or clinical social worker before the CSE meeting.

During the CSE meeting, the results of the FACT (or another type of assessment tool) will be reviewed to develop a clear picture of the ways your child's ADHD (and any learning disabilities) are interfering with school success. This information serves as the basis for the developing of an IEP or 504 Plan. IEPs are developed if there appears to be the need for services by special education teachers; 504 Plans are developed if you and the district are of the opinion that your child could be successful without special education services provided the child is given certain reasonable accommodations. A sample of the kinds of accommodations that are considered reasonable by at least two school districts (Broward County, Florida; Vestal Central School District, New York) follows. Accommodations include modifications in the physical arrangement of the room, lesson presentation, completion of assignments, test taking, organization and behavioral expectations.

Like the FACT, this list of accommodations should be available at the time of your CSE meeting. It is intended to be used as a reference by you and the committee. The goal of the committee is to develop a plan that includes (as needed) instruction by a special education teacher and provision for certain types of accommodations and modifications designed to help your child succeed. Once you and your district are in agreement regarding the plan, a written version of the plan will be submitted to the board of education in

The Functional Assessment Checklist for Teachers (FACT)

Student's Name: _____

Teacher's Name: _____

Date of Rating: _____

Dear: _____

As you are aware, children with attention-deficit/hyperactivity disorder (ADHD) have a health impairment that can adversely affect their functioning at school. To develop comprehensive intervention programs that can promote the success of these children, functional assessment of the child's behavior at school is essential. Your assistance in this process would be greatly appreciated.

The following statements relate to specific abilities that are commonly affected by ADHD. Please read each statement and assign a value using the following scale.

1. Far worse than peers
2. Slightly worse than peers
3. About the same as peers
4. Slightly better than peers
5. Much better than peers

N. Not expected at this age

ORGANIZATION:
_____ Arrives to class on time
_____ Has necessary materials (textbook, paper, etc.)
_____ Brings homework assignments to class
_____ Records homework assignments in planner/agenda
_____ Brings home the materials necessary to complete homework

CLASSROOM FUNCTIONING:
_____ Sits in seat, does not disrupt class with extraneous movements or verbalizations
_____ Follows written directions

The Functional Assessment Checklist for Teachers (FACT) (*Continued*)

_____ Follows verbal directions
_____ Accurately copies notes from chalkboard or overheads
_____ Completes seat work during the allowed time
_____ Takes accurate notes from lectures or instructional presentations
_____ Participates appropriately in class discussions (does not interrupt; stays on topics)

SOCIAL SKILLS:

_____ Maintains eye contact while speaking
_____ Maintains eye contact while listening
_____ Engages in social conversations with peers
_____ Is able to maintain a conversation that is of interest to the other person
_____ Is invited by peers to join social activities
_____ Is involved in school-based extracurricular activities (e.g., sports, music, drama)

AFFECTIVE CONTROL:

_____ Tolerates frustration
_____ Verbally aggressive with peers
_____ Verbally aggressive with staff
_____ Complies with rules
_____ Physically aggressive with peers
_____ Physically aggressive with staff
_____ Seems anxious or worried
_____ Seems sad/depressed

ACADEMIC SKILLS:
Reading:

_____ Reading speed and accuracy
_____ Ability to comprehend the content of passages
_____ Ability to reach conclusions based on inference
_____ Ability to prepare outlines or study guides based on reading of textbook

(continued)

The Functional Assessment Checklist for Teachers (FACT) (*Continued*)

Mathematics:
_____ Knowledge of number facts (addition/subtraction)
_____ Knowledge of multiplication facts
_____ Computational accuracy
_____ Ability to understand word problems and calculate the correct answer

Written Expression:
_____ Writing speed
_____ Writing legibility
_____ Spelling skills
_____ Grammar skills
_____ Ability to write answers requiring a single sentence
_____ Ability to write short essays (one or two paragraphs)
_____ Ability to write compositions (three or more paragraphs)

© Vincent J. Monastra, PhD

---

your child's school district. Once accepted, the provisions in the plan must be followed. Educational law requires that these plans be reviewed (and revised if necessary) at least once per year. In addition, should the plan need revision before the year is completed, it can be reviewed and revised at the written request of the parent or the school.

HOMEWORK

A lot of information was presented to you in this lesson. Before you proceed to the next lesson, take a little time to think about how your child is doing in school. If your son or daughter has ADHD, does

Accommodations Provided in Accordance With Section 504 of the Rehabilitation Act of 1973

Physical Arrangement of the Room:

_____ Seating the student near the teacher

_____ Seating the student near a positive role model

_____ Teacher will stand near the student when giving directions or presenting lessons

_____ Student will be placed away from distracting stimuli (e.g. window, door)

_____ Teacher will increase the distance between the student's desk and classmates' desks

Lesson Presentation:

_____ Pair students to check accuracy of work

_____ Write key points on the board

_____ Provide peer tutoring

_____ Provide peer note-taker

_____ Provide written outline

_____ Allow student to tape record lessons

_____ Have child review key points orally

_____ Use computer-assisted instruction (software, Internet)

_____ Permit student to use word-processing technology to take notes

_____ Make sure directions are understood

_____ Include a variety of activities during each lesson

_____ Divide longer presentations into shorter segments

Assignments and Worksheets:

_____ Give extra time to complete tasks

_____ Simplify complex directions

_____ Hand out worksheets one at a time

_____ Reduce the reading level of the assignments

_____ Require fewer correct responses to achieve grade

_____ Require fewer repetitions of practice work (e.g., spelling lists, math worksheets)

(continued)

Accommodations Provided in Accordance With Section 504 of the Rehabilitation Act of 1973 (*Continued*)

_____ Reduce the number of homework assignments

_____ Allow the student to use voice-recognition software to complete homework

_____ Allow the student to use a word processor or computer to complete written work

_____ Provide structured guides for completing written assignments

_____ Provide study skills training

_____ Shorten assignments; divide work into smaller segments

_____ Do not grade handwriting or spelling (unless a spelling test)

Test Modifications:

_____ Allow extra time to complete tests

_____ Permit test to be taken in a low distraction context

_____ Permit use of assistive technology (tape recorder, voice-recognition software, or word processor) to record answers

_____ Read test items to the student

_____ Permit a scribe to record answers

_____ Read directions to the student; check to determine understanding of directions

_____ Give exam orally

_____ Give take-home tests

_____ Use more objective questions (fewer essay responses)

_____ Give frequent short quizzes, not long exams

_____ Allow periodic "breaks" during testing

_____ Allow periodic interactions with teacher or examiner to promote attention to task

Organization:

_____ Provide peer assistance with organizational skills

_____ Assign homework buddy

_____ Provide extra set of books at home

_____ Send daily or weekly progress reports home, listing specific assignments that were not completed or returned, and defining any behavioral concerns

Accommodations Provided in Accordance With Section 504 of the Rehabilitation Act of 1973 *(Continued)*

_____ Develop a reward system for classroom work and homework completion
_____ Provide the student with a homework assignments notebook
_____ Check accuracy of daily assignment notebook
_____ Prompt the student regarding assignments and materials that need to be brought home
_____ Prompt the student to turn in completed homework

Behavior:
_____ Develop and implement a classroom behavior management system
_____ Praise specific behaviors
_____ Use privileges and rewards for specific behaviors
_____ Make "prudent use" of negative consequences
_____ Keep classroom rules simple and clear
_____ Allow for short breaks between assignments
_____ Use nonverbal cues to help student stay on task
_____ Mark student's correct answers, not mistakes
_____ Permit time out of seat for "movement" (e.g., run errands)
_____ Allow movement that does not distract others
_____ Develop "contracts" with the student
_____ Use time-out procedures
_____ Ignore inappropriate behaviors not drastically outside classroom limits

he or she have an IEP or 504 Plan? If so, how is it working? If your child's grades are still low and have not improved significantly since implementing the IEP or 504 Plan, then revision is needed.

The purpose of educational laws is to make sure that your child is succeeding at school and demonstrating an ability to learn academic material at a level consistent with his or her intelligence. If your child is receiving grades of 65 to 70 because he or she is not completing (or is forgetting to turn in) assignments, the IEP needs to be revised. If your child is failing courses because she or he cannot prepare study guides, the IEP needs to be revised. If your child is being repeatedly disciplined for ADHD behaviors (e.g., unable to complete seat work on time, failure to return homework assignments, speaking out of turn, displaying restlessness while seated), the IEP needs to be revised. Write to the CSE chairperson and get the process started.

Similarly, if your child has been diagnosed with ADHD but is not receiving academic support, now is the time to write a letter to your district's CSE chairperson. Although efforts to motivate students through rewards and punishments are understandable, it is a gross mistake to believe that such strategies alone will overcome the range of functional impairments caused by ADHD. Kids with ADHD need an educational plan that specifically targets their multiple areas of functional impairment. Whereas use of daily and weekly feedback from teachers to parents can help increase student motivation, anyone who understands that ADHD is a health impairment fully recognizes that such reporting of failure does not breed academic success.

We would not expect to help a blind child improve her or his eyesight by withholding privileges or administering punishments. The same holds true for children with other types of health problems, like ADHD. Don't succumb to the notion that the cause of your child's failure is that she or he is hopelessly unmotivated, depressed, or defiant. Don't give away your child's educational rights. Get your child the help he or she deserves!

LESSON 6

KIDS NEED A REASON TO LEARN

During the first five lessons, I spent a lot of time telling you that attention-deficit/hyperactivity disorder (ADHD) is a medical condition, that it is inherited, and that at least some of the symptoms are likely to continue into adulthood. You've read about how medications for ADHD work and how proper nutrition can help your child. You've also learned about attention-training programs that can be used to treat core symptoms of ADHD. However, even though medication, dietary changes, and attention-training programs can help your child's brain "wake up," many problems at home and school will continue without systematic intervention.

Sometimes I think that medicines for ADHD help in the same way that a medicine for blindness might. What I mean is this: Let's say that someone developed a medicine that cured blindness. After a patient took the medicine, she would be able to see. However, she wouldn't know the names of the numerous objects she could now see. The patient wouldn't know how to read printed words or how to "read" facial expressions, among other things.

A similar type of process occurs with ADHD. When a patient is treated with an effective dose of medication, he often feels that he can sit still, pay attention, and concentrate for longer periods of time. However, the medicine does not teach the patient how to take notes in class, search books for facts, prepare study guides, complete outlines and essays, or study for tests. The medicine does not develop a plan so the patient is organized and remembers important aspects of life. The medicine does not create an ability to find the words needed to have conversations that are of interest to other kids (or his parents). The medicine does not help him know how to solve problems that occur at home, at school, or in the neighborhood. That kind of knowledge must be taught and learned.

Earlier in this book, I provided you with a long list of lessons you might want your child to learn. The lessons listed in "What I'd Like My Child to Learn" are those that commonly need to be taught to children with ADHD. Take a few moments to look at that list. As you look at it, remember that some of the lessons will be addressed at school, through the development of an Individualized Education Plan or 504 Accommodation Plan. However, other skills will need to be developed primarily at home. In this lesson, I examine how you can help your child overcome some of the social and academic problems that are part of ADHD.

HOW DO KIDS LEARN NEW SKILLS?

A fair amount is known about the learning process. Here are some basics.

1. *The teacher (in this case, you) needs to select a skill that the child is physically able to learn.* For example, you might be able to teach a 6-year-old to organize his or her belongings by picking up toys after playing. You would not be successful if you asked the same child to organize the garage. So the first question you need to ask yourself when you think about teaching your child is, "Is this skill something that kids within 2 years of my child's age are generally able to do?"

2. The child needs to be attending when you are teaching. This means that to teach your child to learn, you need to make sure that he or she is listening (and looking if you are showing the child something). Because kids with ADHD often listen while looking at other things, this doesn't mean that you have to get into an argument over the need to look at you. It just means that you need to check and make sure the child heard you.

3. Your lesson needs to be brief and to the point. If you make a big preliminary speech about your child's laziness and how frustrated you are and then launch into your directions, chances are that your kid has drifted off. Figure that you have about 10 to 20 seconds to get your message across. So before you sit down with your child, you might want to write down exactly what you want to them to do. If you want your child to pick up all clothes, toys, books, and food wrappers from the floor of her room and put them in a box (for later sorting), then tell her that. Kids with ADHD do not have an internalized model of what a clean bedroom looks like. They need to learn. Similarly, if your child needs to study for a test, it is pointless to tell him, "Go to your room and study." He probably has no idea how to study. Again, you'll need to teach your child or hire a tutor to help him learn how to study (e.g., "Let's look at your chapter review. I'll ask you the questions. If there is any question you can't answer, I'll help you find the information and write the answer down on a piece of paper or index card. You can memorize the facts on each card, and I'll test you to make sure that you know most of them.")

4. The child needs to have a reason for learning. This is a biggie. Without motivation, there is little learning. Think back to your high school or college days. If a teacher told you to read a book chapter or a magazine article before the next class, did you always do it? If my memory is working, I remember that there was always someone in the class who'd ask, "Is this going to be on the test?" or "Are we going to have a quiz on this?" If the teacher said yes, chances are you'd try to read it. If the teacher said no, chances are you wouldn't. Now there was always the chance that you were absolutely fascinated by the subject material (a long shot for most of us) and would read the material because you were interested in it. However, without that type of interest, most of us needed some type of external motivator (e.g., the knowledge that we'd be grounded, lose our driving privileges, or be unable to play sports for our school team if we did poorly on the test).

5. *The child needs to know when he or she needs to perform the skill you are teaching.* Kids with ADHD do not have a great sense of time. Without a specific time requirement, the task will be put into the "later" category, which translates to "any time but now." After you tell a child with ADHD to do something, they will typically return to doing what they were enjoying before you asked. Internally, they say some version of "I'll do that later." This applies to chores, homework, and other "low-likeability" tasks. So for your child to do what you want, you'll have to define when the task needs to be done.

Let's try to apply these realities to teaching the child with ADHD. It is true that your child will need some type of motivating reason to learn and do what he or she has been taught. However, unlike with kids without ADHD, it is important for you to realize that some long-term reward, like a special trip, or punishment or consequence such as being grounded or being dropped from the football team, is not going to work. It is highly unlikely that your child will get all passing grades, turn in all assignments, and not have a single disciplinary referral simply because you offered to take him to Disney World as a reward for that kind of effort over a 10-week marking period. It is equally unlikely that a major turnaround would occur if you grounded your child for days or weeks if she did not pass a test or turn in an assignment or got into trouble at school.

I encourage parents not to use such a "big-bang" approach. Instead, I want you to think about all the "free" pleasures that your child receives every day. Many kids get to watch cable television and have access to literally hundreds of channels. A surprisingly high percentage of kids have endlessly entertaining smartphones. Others are able to play incredibly fascinating games on computers, Wiis, or other video gaming systems. They are able to explore an incredible world of information and communication online. They can go outside and ride their bikes, rollerblade, skateboard, or play soccer, baseball, basketball, football, or other sports. They can build with their Legos. They can play the guitar, the piano, the drums, or other instruments. They can go to karate, scouts, and participate as a member of a sporting team. Instead of offering your kids money, a big event, or some other all-or-nothing type of deal, I want you to begin thinking about how you can use these daily pleasures to motivate your child to learn.

For example, let's say you want your child to learn to keep the floor of the bedroom free of toys, clothing, papers, food, and drinks. You've told your son or daughter hundreds of times to keep the room picked up. It's morning. You wake up and battle to get your child awake, fed, washed, dressed, and out the door. For reasons unknown to you or me, you walk into the bedroom as your child is getting ready. You notice the room is a mess. You hit the roof. You tell your child that because the room isn't picked up, he or she is grounded after school. What is likely to happen now? Big emotional meltdown!

Somehow, you get through that moment, but what about after school? Well, there is little chance that your child will ground him- or herself (because you're working). And because one of the twice-weekly soccer league games is on the schedule that night (and we can't let the team down), the kid gets to play soccer. So even though you've told her or him to pick up the bedroom hundreds of times, made sure you had her or his attention when you said it, and had even shown the child what a clean room looks like, there is no reason for your child to do what you've asked. After all, the child was able to come home after school, have a snack, watch television, play video games, talk with a friend, and maybe even get homework done (a long shot). To top it off, tonight there is a game. The child may think, "Why pick up my room?" (even if he or she somehow remembers the need to do so). More likely, the child will think "I'll do it later," but the cool thing is that "later" is "anytime but now." So it doesn't get done.

Another essential truth to keep in mind is that your child is unlikely to be inspired to do what you want because of some internalized motivational source (e.g., "It will make Mom happy"; "I've got to learn to be organized so I can be successful when I go to Harvard"). Without an immediate, concrete reason that can't be ignored, you'll harp on the same issue forever. My suggestion for the kid with the messy room is some variation of the following: "Billy, after school you'll need to pick up the toys, clothes, and junk off the floor and put them in this bag before you can go to soccer. If the room is not picked up by the time I get home, you'll have that job, plus another one to do. We'll go to soccer when they're both done. So it's up to you, son." I might also add, "I can give you a call to remind you" or help him set up some type of prompt to remind himself (e.g., on his smart phone). The key element here is that your child needs to comply with your requests to earn the right to do something that she or he has been getting for free. A lesson I share with my patients with ADHD is that their parents are trying to help them grow up. When they were babies, everything was free. Now that they are growing up and want to do "big kid" stuff, they have to earn it. In life, you get what you work for. Moms and dads need to help kids learn that lesson.

The other thing you need to keep in mind is that you don't have to bribe your kid with toys, trips to the mall, videos, video games, or money to motivate him or her to learn the lessons you are trying to teach. Instead, as you think about your child's day and all the freebies he or she receives regardless of whether the child listens to you or not, you'll come to realize that there is a world of opportunity to use those types of activities to inspire better effort. Instead of bribing, we will examine ways to organize your child's day so that he or she needs to earn life's daily pleasures. There are few freebies and no sacred cows (not even Little League baseball games) that can't be postponed until the task is done. In the next lesson, I talk about the systematic use of daily pleasures to motivate and the use of a procedure I call "Time Stands Still." More on that in a little bit.

6. *Kids learn best from teachers who are respectful and show that they care.* Before I discuss strategies such as Time Stands Still and the use of daily pleasures, I want to take a minute to emphasize one last piece in the learning process. It has to do with the characteristics of the teacher. Think back on your childhood. Whom do you remember as an effective teacher? For many people, a somewhat demanding teacher who was firm but fair may come to mind. This person may not have had a great sense of humor. Probably, this teacher gave you a lot of homework. But there was something about this teacher that made you work a little harder. Maybe you had the sense that he or she liked or respected you. Maybe this teacher complimented you on your abilities. Maybe the teacher took a little time after class to explain lessons to you. Maybe she or he had a kind word for you when the teacher saw you in the hall. Maybe this teacher took an interest in your activities. The bottom line is that you had the sense that this teacher cared about you. And you responded. This type of teacher model can be useful in teaching kids with ADHD, whether at school or at home.

Other effective teachers have a great sense of humor and can teach complex ideas in enjoyable ways. These teachers are highly creative and fun. They hold the attention of students because they are entertaining. Just like the preacher who cracks a few jokes or shares personal experiences, these teachers help kids learn because most people pay closer attention after a refreshing bit of humor or a good story. If you have a good sense of humor and can find the fun in teaching mundane things like brushing teeth or picking up a room, you might be able to use this type of teaching strategy.

A third type of teaching style uses a lot of criticism, threats, and punishment. When a child makes a mistake, forgets, or fails to comply with a parental request, she or he is spoken to harshly, put down, and receives some type of punishment (e.g., a restriction to the bedroom for the remainder of the day or the loss of a planned activity). Believe it or not, I have even interviewed kids who have told me that they "lost Christmas" because their rooms were a mess and they were fighting with their brothers and sisters too much. In these families, the parents actually threw out the Christmas presents in an effort to teach their children to obey. Although the memory of the loss of Christmas present remained a disturbing one to these children, the parents' use of this harsh approach failed to stop the fighting or get the rooms clean. Remember, regardless of how severely a parent (or teacher) criticizes or punishes a child with ADHD, such punitive approaches fail miserably with these children. Instead, children with ADHD either become highly aggressive in response to this type of approach or simply get distracted by some other entertaining aspect of their world and quickly forget even what they're being punished for.

As your child's primary teacher when it comes to learning those personal skills needed to succeed in life, it is up to you to decide what type of teacher you will be. For the most part, I think people tend to learn more from someone we feel cares about and respects us. The same is true with our kids. Children need to know that their parents (or other caregivers) love them and think they are an OK person. It will be important for you to communicate this to your child, day to day, as you work on teaching new skills.

HOMEWORK

During the coming week, I want you to begin thinking about a couple of topics. First, consider the amount of time you get to spend saying something nice to or doing something nice with your kid. Here's what I mean by *nice*. For at least 15 minutes each day, I'd like you to be in a room with your child and actually interact with him or her (talking, hanging out, or doing something enjoyable) without asking questions, giving directions, or correcting. Now this may sound simple, but check out what happens most times you are near your child. Chances are that you ask questions or tell your child to do something or stop doing something. I am asking you to be in the same room without doing any of that, at least once a day, every day, for 15 minutes. That's what I mean by *nice*.

The reason this is important is that by the time many kids with ADHD reach age 8 years, they start to react to your presence with indifference or a bit of dread. If the only time your kids hear you call their name is when they are in trouble or need to do some kind of chore, why listen? Letting your children know that you are interested in being with them for reasons other than bossing them around is a good place to start. Your children need to feel that you actually like being their parent, that you love and want to be with them, and that they are far more than just a burden to you.

The second task has to do with taking a closer look at the reasons your child continues to do things you want her or him to stop (or fails to do the tasks you want the child to start). Pull out your "What I'd Like My Child to Learn" list. Select around six lessons that you want your child to learn. Write each down on a separate piece of paper. Now do the following.

Think about what it takes for a child to learn. For each of the lessons you have been trying to teach your child, ask yourself the following:

1. Am I looking for my kid to do something beyond his or her abilities (is this something that kids within 2 years of his or her age are generally able to do)?
2. Do I have my child's attention when I'm trying to teach?
3. Have I figured out a way to teach the lesson in 10 to 20 seconds?
4. Have I shown or told my child what I want her or him to do (or stop doing)?
5. Is there a reason for my child to do what I want?
6. Am I speaking to my son or daughter in a way that demonstrates caring?

As you think about those lessons your child has not yet learned, you'll probably find that some of the reasons are found in the answers to these questions. Another common reason for feeling as though you have failed as a parent is because there are so many things going wrong that you don't know where to start. I'll help you with that as we go through these lessons. For now, just begin to think about the kinds of lessons you want to teach and the importance of developing a specific plan. In the next few lessons, I'll talk specifically about ways to help your child become more organized, able to complete responsibilities, learn behavioral and emotional control, and develop effective problem-solving skills. To help you begin this process, I have included a guide at the end of this lesson for you to use.

One last thought before we move on. Many parents who I work with beat themselves up because their children have so many problems. I'm hoping you haven't forgotten all the talk in earlier lessons about how ADHD is a real disorder and how it is a medical condition that you didn't cause. It is true that there are a lot of lessons you'll want to teach your child, but once you have taken the steps to address the physical causes of your child's problems (through medication, biofeedback, or other interventions), you will have a child who can be taught. If you can plan on teaching your child one new skill every week or so, you'll be amazed how much can change in a year!

Guide for Teaching Skills to Your Child

1. Write down one lesson you want to teach your child.

_____

_____

2. Is this something that kids within 2 years of your child's age are able to do? If no, pick another lesson.

_____

3. When are you going to do your "teaching"? Pick a time, and a place with few distractions.

_____

4. Have you told or shown your child what you wanted him or her to do (or stop doing)? Remember the 10-second rule!

_____

5. What will happen if your child does what you want? Make sure that your child knows this.

_____

_____

6. What will happen if your child doesn't do what you want? Make sure that your child knows this, too.

_____

_____

© Vincent J. Monastra, PhD

LESSON 7

YOU'LL GET LOST WITHOUT A LESSON PLAN

As I begin parenting classes at my clinic, I am often struck by how tired and drained the parents of my patients look. I treat a wide range of patients, from 4-year-old children to adults in their 70s. However, most of my patients are school-age children. This means that most of the parents in my classes have essentially had to function as their child's frontal lobe for more than a decade. They needed to remain highly vigilant to help their child fulfill responsibilities. They had to be ever-mindful of their child's whereabouts to protect the child from harm. They spent hours calming their child when he or she was uncontrollably distraught over events that others would shrug off. They exhausted themselves as they tried to convince their child not to act on aggressive impulses when frustrated. By the time these parents come to see me, they have tried pretty much everything others have suggested. They are tired and frustrated.

This book follows the outline of the program in use at my clinic, and you and I are now seven sessions into the book (or "class"). We still haven't set up a single *token economy* (a home program in which kids earn points or chips to buy fun time or rewards). There are no star charts plastered on the refrigerator door. The kids are not receiving stickers, dimes, or dollars for each good behavior they exhibit. Yet you parents are beginning to look a bit more ener-gized. The reason? Some significant events have occurred.

For example, if you are following my plan, your child has been evaluated by a physician to make sure that she or he does not have any other medical problem that can cause symptoms of inattention, hyperactivity, and impulsivity. At least 10% of children have been diagnosed with other medical problems that have been contribut-ing to these symptoms (most commonly vitamin D deficiencies, allergies, visual tracking or convergence disorders, and psycho-active substance abuse), and treatments for these problems have been initiated. Nutritional evaluations are complete, and dietary prob-lems (most often lack of protein at breakfast and lunch) have been identified. Efforts to improve your child's diet have begun. Sleep problems have been recognized, and your child is now getting a suf-ficient amount of sleep to help him or her pay attention during the day. Because most of my patients are treated with medication for attention-deficit/hyperactivity disorder (ADHD; in combination with attention-training programs), I would also expect that your child's physician has taken steps to identify an effective type and dose of medication and that your child is beginning to respond.

In addition, parents should have written letters to the chairper-son of their school district's Committee on Special Education. If so, educational evaluations are now in process at school for the child. Some children may have started to receive academic support at this time. At home, parents are trying to spend some playtime with their children. In short, you have begun to set the stage for teaching at home.

In some ways, I compare initial efforts at my clinic to work in an emergency department at a hospital. The patient comes in, there is a great degree of risk, and the first task is to stabilize the patient's medical condition. This is what we have done so far: stabilized the situation so you can begin to teach your child some important skills. It is now time to develop your lesson plans.

PARENTS AS TEACHERS

As I mentioned before, my hope is that you can fight the tendency to get overwhelmed by the number of lessons that you want to teach your child. Parenting requires a lesson plan. Like any other teacher, you need to realize that you should teach one lesson at a time. I encourage my parents to remember that there are 52 weeks in a year. That means if you only teach one lesson a week, you will have taught 52 lessons that year. However, to be honest, I haven't been involved in too many situations in which the number of significant problems exceeded a dozen or so. By the time parents are comfortable with the idea of systematically using daily pleasures to motivate and have experienced success with the first six lessons, teaching begins to move forward with much less effort. So, as we continue with your lesson plan, it is important to realize that it is better to work on a few lessons at a time and to remember that your child will need a reason to learn. This will be as true for other children in your family as for your child with ADHD.

When parents consider ways to motivate their children with ADHD, the use of *reinforcers* (e.g., objects such as money, toys, or videos, or activities such as playing outside, visiting a friend, use of the family computer or computer games) typically comes to mind. However, parents and counselors who treat children with ADHD have learned that it isn't easy to use objects or activities to motivate kids with ADHD to complete daily tasks like getting up in the morning, eating a nutritious breakfast, brushing teeth, getting dressed, making it out the door to catch the school bus on time, cooperating with the teacher, completing assigned work, bringing home and completing homework, listening to (and doing) what Mom and Dad ask them to do, getting along with brothers and sisters, helping with chores such as cleaning their room or other areas in the house, and going to bed without a fight. Unlike other kids, who might have little problem completing 90% of these tasks, kids with ADHD need motivation to complete nearly all of them.

If your child doesn't have ADHD and does 90% of these tasks anyway, but leaves his or her room a mess, then you could easily use a reinforcer such as not going out after school to play until the room is cleaned to inspire the child. The child who does not have ADHD would most likely come home and quickly put her or his clothes in drawers (or the closet), pick up trash off the floor, and put toys in some type of container or on a shelf. Now I'm not saying the job would be done perfectly. However, those areas needing further work (e.g., the closet where everything was piled into) would be pointed out and the child informed that the closet also needed to be organized. Although the kid without ADHD would not be too happy about the parent's actions, it is highly unlikely that the child would have a meltdown and trash the room. A kid with ADHD might.

Let's look at how this room-cleaning requirement would work for the child with ADHD. The child comes home but probably forgets that he or she needs to clean the room. If you are home, you'll need to remind the child, because odds are he or she is already playing. So you have to interrupt playtime (and listen to the arguing and pleading) and direct the child to go clean up. More debate and arguing are likely to come next. Finally, when the child gets to the bedroom she or he will probably get distracted and start playing with something else. Old toys, pieces of paper, and other memorabilia can be fascinating when the alternative is to begin putting away clothes, toys, or other things.

After a half hour or so of thinking that your child is busily cleaning the room, you check in to discover that nothing has happened. So you remind the child to get started or he or she can't go outside to play. However, by now it's getting dark anyway. So maybe you threaten that the child won't be able to go out tomorrow. Or maybe you threaten to ground your child from television, the smartphone, or video games. Regardless of what you do, this is a hopeless situation that is going nowhere fast. And this is only one of numerous tasks you want your child to complete on a daily basis.

Because doctors and counselors have long recognized that children with ADHD do not usually respond well to the kinds of reinforcers typically used by parents, more systematic approaches have been developed. One involves the development of home behavior charts or programs (sometimes *called point systems, star charts,* or *token economies*) that chart the specific kinds of tasks the child is expected to complete and the specific kinds of objects and activities that he or she can earn by completing them. If the child completes the desired task (e.g., doing homework) or acts in certain desired ways (e.g., not arguing or playing cooperatively), he or she can earn a reward (e.g., money or a toy) or permission to do some activity (e.g., play a game or visit a friend). If the child does not complete the task or act in the desired way, he or she does not earn the reward. Such programs have been studied for some time and, when well thought out, can be helpful in promoting the development of children, including some of those who have ADHD.

However, because many parents I work with have ADHD themselves or are overwhelmed by the prospects of developing a comprehensive home charting plan, it is often easier to use a simpler *Work for Play* type of program, which was developed at our clinic. In the Work for Play program, the day is divided into four time periods (before school, at school, before dinner, after dinner). The child needs to complete certain tasks to earn the privilege to engage in any recreational activity during each time period.

In Work for Play, if the child does what is required, he or she can play for that time period. If she or he does not do what is required, a procedure that I call "Time Stands Still" is used. In this process, the child does not have permission to engage in any activity other than the one required by the parent. His or her life is on hold until the child complies. The longer he or she delays (and defies his or her parents or says upsetting things), the more the child will need to do to make up for these actions.

This process is quite different from the familiar time out because there is no time limit on the punishment. In Time Stands Still, the child needs to comply with parental requests and make up for disrespectful actions before he or she can play. The longer he or she delays, the more the child will need to do to make up. This is intended to place responsibility clearly on the child's shoulders and to teach the lesson that people need to apologize and make amends when they do things that upset or hurt others. In time out, children may be placed in a chair for 1 minute for every year of age, for example, if they do not comply with a parent's request. Supposedly, that 5 minutes in the chair will motivate a child to stop bopping his sister on the head, for example. If you have a kid with ADHD, you already know that this doesn't work.

Now if your child defies you, does not do what you ask, and plays anyway (without permission), she or he will need to apologize, do some type of corrective activity (to make up), and obey the parent's request. If the defiance occurs before school, the child cannot play after school until she or he apologizes, does some type of corrective activity, and complies with parental requests. Let's take a few minutes and see how each approach works.

Home Behavior Charts

Most parents who attend my classes have heard something about using charts in teaching children with ADHD. Sometimes the words *token economy* are used. Sometimes these charts will be called *point systems, color charts,* or *star charts.* Dr. Harvey Parker, a specialist in creating such programs, uses the term *home behavior chart.* He has published a manual to help parents create these plans (www.

addwarehouse.com). Let me show you a sample program published by Dr. Parker. It describes the skills that Mr. and Mrs. Jones would like their 10-year-old son, Robert, to "Start" as well as the behaviors that these parents want Robert to "Stop." Reasons for learning these parental lessons are listed as "Rewards." Let's take a look at Robert's chart.

Looking at Robert's Home Behavior Chart, his parents wanted their son to wake up by 7:30 a.m., walk the dog, put his schoolbooks back in his bag, clean his bedroom, do his homework, brush his teeth, and jot down notes if he answered the phone. They would award him points for any test or paper returned with a grade of *A* or *B* and give bonus points for completed term papers. These are hardly unreasonable requests. His folks also wanted him to stop butting in, yelling in the house, fighting, taking things without asking permission, coming home late, and leaving the house without permission. Also pretty typical requests. To inspire Robert to learn these skills, his parents were offering typical types of rewards and privileges, such as video game time, television time, the privilege of going outside, staying up later, sleeping over with friends, and certain purchases (e.g., music downloads or baseball cards). So how did Robert do?

Well, on Sunday, he earned 7 points but lost 6 for butting in, which means that he could "buy" none of the available rewards. Now this could be a major problem. I'm sure you've tried preventing your child from enjoying television, video games, or playing outside. That creates a war zone in your house. In addition, once children know there is nothing they can do to earn what they want, they have much less reason to do what you want. So if you choose to use a Home Behavior Chart, you need to think of ways for your child to "get out of jail," so to speak. For example, on your chart you might want to have a *Start Behavior* called *Makes Up* or *Makes Amends*. I like to have these in home programs because it means that the child has a chance to earn some privilege by apologizing and doing some type

Robert's Home Behavior Chart

START	VALUE	SUN.	MON.	TUES.	WED.	THURS.	FRI.	SAT.
WAKES AT 7:30	2		2		2	2	2	2
WALKS DOG	2		2		2	2	2	2
BOOKS IN BAG	1		1	1		1	1	1
CLEAN BEDRM	2		2	2	2		2	2
HOMEWORK	3	3	3	3	3	3		3
BRUSH TEETH	1@	3	2	3	3	3	3	3
WRITE NOTES	1	1	1		1	1		1
MARKS A OR B	2		2	2		2	2	
BONUS PAPER	10							
TOTAL		7	15	11	13	14	12	12

****

STOP BEHAVIORS

	VALUE	SUN.	MON.	TUES.	WED.	THURS.	FRI.	SAT.
BUTTS IN	−5	−5						
YELLS	−5		−5					
FIGHT	−10							−5

	COST							
TAKES STUFF	−10							
HOME LATE	−10							
LEAVE HOUSE	−10							
TOTAL		−5	−5		−10	−10		−5
ROBERT EARNS		2	10	11	3	14	12	2
REWARDS	**COST**							
GAME 30 MIN	3		3	3	3		3	3
T.V. 30 MIN	3		3	3	3		3	6
PLAY OUTSIDE	3							
STAY UP LATER	4							4
SWEET SNACK	3			3				
BUY CARDS	10					10		
SLEEPOVER	20							
BUY CD	30							
USED		0	6	9	6	10	6	13
LEFT		2	6	8	5	9	15	9

of action to make amends. I'm big on saying, "If you mess up, you need to make up."

Now look at how Robert did on Monday. Looks like a much better day. He earned 15 points but lost 5 for yelling, which left 10 to spend. He chose to play a video game for 30 minutes and watch television for 30 minutes. Sounds like a nice day on paper, until reality sets in. Have you ever tried to stop a kid who was playing a video game after only a half hour? Maybe I'm living in a really warped part of the world, but the kids who come into my clinic are none too happy if they have to stop playing a game after 30 minutes. They ignore their parents and keep playing. They plead, beg, whine, or throw a tantrum. If Robert did that, he'd lose 5 points for yelling, 5 more for fighting, and quickly be in the hole.

So on a day in which Robert did pretty much everything his folks wanted (woke up, walked the dog, picked up his books, cleaned his room, did his homework, brushed his teeth twice, jotted down notes, and received an *A* or *B* on a school paper), he ended up pretty frustrated and probably in a bit of trouble with his folks. For all his efforts, he was only able to play a video game for 30 minutes and watch television for 30 minutes. Most kids with ADHD get to do that anyway. To top it off, he probably got angry with his parents when they told him to stop playing his video game. What could be done to make this work out better for Robert and his parents?

One of the most important parts of setting up a home behavior chart or token economy is to run some simulations of how your "new world" is going to play out. On paper, Robert's program looks pretty good: not too many lessons to be learned, nice things to earn, clearly laid out.

Now run some simulations. In the world Robert's parents created, Robert needs to earn 3 points to watch television or play a video game for 30 minutes. OK, let's say he's a bear to wake up, refuses to walk the dog, fails to pick up his books (you grab them from the four corners of the house), and leaves his room a mess. However, he brushes his teeth twice (2 points), gets a *B* on last night's math homework (2 points), and does his homework tonight (3 points). He earns 7 points and gets an hour's worth of play. How does that sound to you? Probably not too good. To me, as Robert's doctor, I'm not happy either. In his parents' program, he can basically ignore many of their rules and still end up the day doing what he likes. Not a good outcome.

If I revised this program, I would add a Start Behavior like "does what mom or dad asks the first time" (offering 1 to 2 points per time). In fact, that's a mainstay in almost every home behavior chart I work on. I'd also add, "ignores or refuses a mom or dad request" to the Stop Behaviors (docking the child 5–10 points each time). One other Start Behavior I'd add is "apologizes and makes up" (earning 1–3 points) to give the child a chance to get back into the reward game.

A final recommendation is the elimination of the carryover option. As you look at Robert's program, his parents are allowing their son to save points and use them another day. When I use these types of programs, I require kids to use all of their points each day. That way, parents won't get into the situation in which the child has saved enough points to be able to do various fun things while ignoring their rules.

If parents would still like to motivate their child by offering a weekly big-ticket item (like a sleep over or a trip to the movies), they can set weekly targets. For example, if a child could earn a total of 100 points for the school week (5 days), then she or he would qualify for a weekend reward on the basis of this effort. I use 90% (90 points) as an A-effort week that can earn a top-quality reward (e.g., an overnight at a friend's house, $5–$10 allowance); 80% to 89% (B) earns a lesser quality reward (e.g., movie or video game rental).

My experience in using home behavior charts is that they can be helpful if they are well thought out. That's why I encourage you to do some dry runs of your program before you put it into action. Otherwise, it can be a disaster. Here is one of my more memorable disaster stories.

I was working with a family who had two children diagnosed with ADHD. Just like Robert's folks, they had a list of Start Behaviors (pick up, do chores, complete homework, and so on) and used a variety of rewards (game time, television time, play outside, etc.). One of their rewards involved the use of money (the kids could earn $1 per point—these folks had some serious bucks!). Of all the things that they wanted their boys to do, the most important was to get along and not fight. They really, really, really wanted their sons to stop fighting. So, the most valued Start Behavior was "gets along with brother" (meaning no physical fighting and no teasing). The boys could earn 25 points per day simply for not fighting. Guess what happened?

After a couple of days, the boys woke up to the realization that they could basically ignore their parents as long as they just made sure they didn't fight *in front of their parents*. So they'd earn their 25 points for not fighting, cash it in for money and the right to go outside and do their fighting (as needed) away from home. They'd also politely tell their parents that they really didn't feel like doing their chores or homework and remind them that they still planned on watching television because they had earned it by not fighting. Needless to say, this program was changed pretty quickly.

It is important to realize that when you start one of these programs, you are creating a kind of bartering program or economy in your home. Take a moment to think about what the rules are in your home. What does your child need to do to earn television time, video game time, or the right to go to soccer practice or play outside? Anything? For many families I work with, the child is so impulsive, hyperactive, and emotionally explosive that the parents shy away from confrontation with the child. In those homes, the child gets hundreds of reminders and prompts during the day, the parents spend hours debating to get their child to cooperate and in the end still allow the child to play, watch television, or go to their sporting or other events. If children are to learn the lessons they need to succeed in life, they need to learn that in life we get what we earn. There are no free rides. So if they want to play outside, watch television, or go to their event after school, they need to earn it, either by doing what they are supposed to do or by making efforts to make amends if they have messed up.

In a similar manner, I work with a number of parents who provide a rich environment for their child. A daughter may have her own television set, with a DVD and video game system set up in the bedroom, access to a computer with Internet connection, and can visit with friends as she talks on her personal phone ("Mom, everyone has an iPhone or Droid"). She may play on a soccer team, attend karate, take music lessons, and be active in a 4-H club. Now these parents can try to motivate their child by saying, "OK, no television or video games tonight."

But if they turn around and take her to Mickie D's for an early dinner (because it's soccer night), and she plays soccer with her friends, gets a soda and snack at the refreshment stand (because she's so exhausted from practice), then ends up going home and crashing into bed to read her favorite fantasy book, do you think she really cares that she missed out on TV time? After all, she wasn't going to be able to watch it anyway.

If you decide to use a charting type of program, try to minimize the number of "sacred cows." I define a *sacred cow activity* as one that the child gets to do regardless of his or her actions. My recommendation is that parents eliminate the sacred cow concept. I usually get some tough looks from the fathers in the parenting class who are

Little League coaches. They tell me that their child has a responsibility to his teammates and can't let them down. I'm not suggesting that you ground your child from the big game because he didn't clean up his room, forgot to walk the dog, or yelled at his brother. What I am recommending is that if your child did that, then the child needs to earn the right to play ball by doing some kind of corrective action before the game. Being attentive to that part of the process is an essential ingredient in making home behavior programs successful.

This Sounds Too Complicated to Me. Isn't There a Simpler Way?

Yes! As I mentioned, charting strategies have a lot of positive ingredients. Parents clearly define what they want their children to learn. Children are informed about the program and know what they need to do and what they can earn. Rewards and privileges are clearly spelled out so kids have a reason to learn the lessons their parents are trying to teach. However, the most glaring problem with these programs is that they can be overwhelming to those parents who have attention deficits themselves. In my classes many, if not most, of the people attending have organizational problems, whether it's because of their own ADHD, the demands of their work schedule, or the stress of being a single parent raising children alone, for example. The charting approach simply overwhelms them.

Let's go back to Robert's chart. His folks wanted him to do certain tasks and stop other behaviors. They created a point system and used that to motivate him. However, their plan required real diligence, a record-keeping system, and a lot of detail. It also required a parent to be present after school, which is challenging if you're a single parent with a full-time job or if both parents work full time. A simpler approach is the Work for Play plan that we use at my clinic.

What Do You Mean by Work for Play?

A long time ago, when I was growing up in the suburbs of Philadelphia, I lived on a dead-end street that contained about 50 row homes (the current term is *townhouse*). The houses were all connected. In fact, at night we could talk with our buddies next door through the air vents. There were seemingly hundreds of kids playing on my one block. It was great! And highly motivating. Parents in my neighborhood weren't using point charts or star charts. They used a variation of the Work for Play plan. I'll give you an example.

Like Robert, kids whose parents were using the Work for Play plan had morning chores and responsibilities. They had to wake up, get washed, dressed, pick up their room, grab breakfast, and be ready for school on time. If they did, great! The child would get a little time to watch television. When the child came home after school, he or she would have some type of simple chore and quickly head out to play (or watch television).

However, if you gave your mom a hard time and didn't do what you needed to do, there was no morning television. When you came home from school, you did the morning chores that you had failed to do, then you did your after-school chore, plus some extra duties (e.g., dusting, cleaning a bathroom), and then you could go outside or watch television. You needed to be home on time for dinner (or homework). Finally, each child had responsibilities after dinner (e.g., homework, washing the dishes, getting ready for bed) before she or he could watch television or play games.

This type of approach created an unspoken kind or organization. The child had certain responsibilities that needed to be finished before he or she could earn the rewards or privileges available at that time of day. To earn play time, the child had certain tasks. If the child didn't complete them, she or he was given extra tasks that needed to be completed, in addition to what the child failed to do, before play time could begin. The process included a morning routine, a during-school routine, an after-school routine, and an evening routine. Instead of creating a situation in which the child was grounded or was unable to earn play time because he or she was "bad" in the morning, the child needed to correct the behavior, do what was required, and then make up for the misbehavior by apologizing and doing extra tasks.

The simplicity of this type of plan is often attractive to the parents in my class. It also is easy to implement if your child goes to a day-care location after school. As with the charting approach, parents are asked to select goals from the What I'd Like My Child to Learn list. The next step is dividing these goals into morning, during-school, after-school, and evening periods and deciding which the child needs to do during each period to earn their playtime.

What If My Child Refuses to Do What I Ask?

A common event for parents of kids with ADHD is the emotional upheaval that occurs when their children are asked to do something that they do not want to do. This could be a chore, homework, or making up for misbehavior. Battle lines will be drawn quickly. The children with ADHD may start yelling, kicking, throwing things, running out of the room, pounding on walls, and so on. Parents initially try to be reasonable but eventually resort to threats and punishments. In these situations, I encourage parents to use three strategies: Time Stands Still, positive practice, and positive punishment.

TIME STANDS STILL. As I discussed earlier, Time Stands Still is different from grounding or other types of punishments. It can be used with children from preschool through high school. It requires that children do what parents have requested before they can earn any privilege (or take part in any enjoyable activity). Until the child complies with the request, his or her life is on hold—time stands still. Or as I say to my older teenage patients, "You go up to the ATM machine and the machine won't give you any money until you enter the correct code. In this case, the correct code is doing what your parents ask."

This means that if your child wants to watch a favorite show, go to a friend's house, go to a game or practice, or do anything other than sit around and read, the child will first need to do what you asked. In this situation, if children start to get upset about being grounded, a parent needs to correct any perception that they have of being grounded. They're not. They can go to a friend's, go to the game, and so on, as soon as they do what you ask. Their life is simply on hold, but they are in control of the situation. The longer they delay, the longer they have to wait to play.

Children will also need to be aware that the longer they delay, the more they make their parents' lives difficult (by yelling, calling names, etc.), and the more effort their parents have to exert to get them to do what is requested of them, the more the children will have to do to get to play. If they balk and delay for 30 minutes or so, with parents having to spend 30 minutes trying to calm them down and convincing them to do what they have been asked, the children will need to do something to make up and give back a bit of energy to their parent. The idea is that if you drain someone of energy, you need to do something to pay that person back. For example, if your child yells at you, calls you names, or uses vulgar language, he or she will need to learn other strategies for expressing frustration. We'll talk more about that in the next lesson.

POSITIVE PRACTICE. Of all of the strategies we've learned from research on reinforcement, the use of *positive practice* is one of the most widely ignored but most powerful approaches. Positive practice simply requires children to practice doing what it is that you asked them to do. So if they balked over taking out the garbage from the kitchen, they would first need to apologize for giving you a hard time and then practice obeying you when you ask them to help. Thus, instead of simply the one task (take out the garbage), you could ask your child to go to the trash baskets in the bathroom, basement, or any other place you have a little basket, gather the trash, and put it in the outside garbage can. The reality is that if you do not do what Mom or Dad asks, then you will still end up doing that task, plus several others to practice doing it the right way. Typically kids learn this lesson pretty quickly.

Now, your attitude during all of this is pretty important too. What you want your child to learn is the simple truth that it's wise to listen to and obey your parents. Firm, loving calmness gets this across far better than "You little snot. You're such a lazy bum. I'm not your slave. All you do is sit around and watch TV and expect me to do everything. So, forget it. You can just figure out another way to get to practice because I'm sick and tired of your attitude. And if you keep it up, you'll be grounded for the weekend!"

Instead, some version of "In our family, we all pitch in and help" is likely to work a lot better. So you could remind your child of that and add your version of "I'd suggest that you hustle on and get the trash out. You know the deal—the longer you wait, the more you'll have to do to make up for it, right? So let's get started."

POSITIVE PUNISHMENT. The last step in addressing what might be called disobedience involves *positive punishment*. It's the technical term for what we all call making up or making amends. In positive punishment, your child will be required to do something to make up for balking at responsibilities. It's not the same as simply doing what was asked in the first place. It's not the same as doing something similar to what he or she didn't do after that. It involves doing something nice for your mom or dad to make up. It's what people do when they say something that's hurtful or make someone else's life harder.

Let's go back to our story of the child who made a big deal out of taking out the trash. After they said "I'm sorry" (the real version, not some half-baked version), did what you asked, and then practiced obeying you and doing some extra chores, there is one more step: making amends. So in our story, after the extra practice, your child will need to do something that says "I'm sorry" to give you back a little of the energy you lost or make up for the time it took for you to get him or her to do the right thing. This could translate to making a snack for you, playing or singing a song for you, writing a list of the things he or she appreciates about you, getting you a cold drink, or something else you'd like.

You maybe noticed that none of these strategies involves being mean. It's all about teaching lessons without triggering a battle. Face it, children are not likely to learn anything from a 30-minute fight with parents over picking up if parents yell, scream, call them all sorts of names, threaten them, take away their favorite stuff, or banish them to their room. Eventually, they'll storm off to the room, thinking Mom or Dad is just a jerk and not learning anything about how families are intended to work. In contrast, positive punishment should help them think twice about not obeying the first time.

To recap, when your child is not obeying, the three strategies I recommend are Time Stands Still, positive practice, and positive punishment. One of the things I like about our approach is that the child is never backed into a corner. Kids with ADHD tend to get aggressive when they are told they have messed up and there is nothing they can do to get what they want. During the period of agitation, they can say and do some hurtful things. If parents stick to their guns and persist in denying their child what is wanted because the child didn't earn it or misbehaved, they are often in for a couple of hours of misery. At the end of it, the parent will often end up doing something to cheer up the child, which in essence negates the effect of the punishment.

With the plan outlined here, children effectively determine how long they will be denied the opportunity to do what they wanted to do. Their actions will also determine the kinds of actions needed to make up. I've learned that kids with ADHD have an incredibly well-developed sense of fairness. It is not hard to teach the idea that they control the duration of their punishment or that they will need to make up for disobedience and hurtful actions. They know what it feels like to be hurt. They also learn pretty quickly that they have no one to blame but themselves if they are delayed in doing something that they like.

HOMEWORK

At this point, I want you to decide which teaching strategy you'd like to begin using. I discussed charting approaches and Work for Play plans, plus Time Stands Still, apologies, and making amends (positive practice and positive punishment). All can be useful, and your choice depends on your style. If you are a person who prefers written contracts and who is fairly well organized, charting may work. If you have difficulties remembering details and tend to be disorganized, the Work for Play plan, combined with Time Stands Still, apologies, positive practice and positive punishment may work a lot better for you. Decide on one.

Next, select your goals from the What I'd Like My Child to Learn list. As I said at the beginning of this lesson, keep it simple. Start with a few goals (six or so) and expand from there. Usually, parents will select a group of goals to begin with and link privileges and rewards to those behaviors. You can use a point system, or you can divide the day into four parts, tell your child what is needed to earn free time for each time period, and take it from there. However, with either approach, it is important to remember that outrageous behaviors (yelling, hitting, screaming, defying) must always be part of the program. In other words, it's fine if you want to reward your child for doing chores or homework, but if the child calls you a name or hits you or a sibling, for example, then she or he will need to perform some type of corrective behavior. It's also important to remember that if you are trying to teach a child not to yell, scream, hit, or be sarcastic, modeling such behaviors isn't going to help. That's pretty much like giving your child a lecture on the health risks of cigarette use while smoking.

After you decide on the type of parenting strategy and select your initial goals, sit down and do several dry runs with another adult. Review what your child needs to do to earn privileges. Make sure it makes sense to you before you tell your child. When you inform your child, let him or her know that your decision was made because he or she is no longer a little kid. Your child needs to hear some version of the following:

> When you were a baby, you might get what you wanted by crying, yelling, and pounding. That was because there wasn't any other way for you to let us know what you needed. Now, you're a lot older, and one of my jobs as your parent is to teach you other ways to get what you want in life. Because part of growing up is learning that you need to earn what you want, we're going to start doing that in our home. Here's how it will work.

If you have more than one child, this lesson is not to be limited to your child with ADHD. If you are developing a plan for your child with ADHD, you should decide on one for your other child or children as well. Their program may include different lessons because they don't have ADHD. However, because most of us need to learn something, I am certain you will be able to decide on lessons that you'd like each of your children to learn.

LESSON 8

TEMPERAMENT MAY BE INHERITED, BUT EMOTIONAL CONTROL IS LEARNED

Now that you have selected the lessons you want your child to learn, an obvious question is staring you in the face. What do you do when your child has a huge tantrum because he or she doesn't like your lesson plan. Let's be honest: Most kids are not going to thank you for teaching them how to organize their rooms, complete their homework, get to bed on time, or eat a healthy variety of foods. There will be times when your child rages about the unfairness of life or broods about how he or she "never gets to do anything," "wish I was dead," "wish someone else was my parent." Although some kids will have lots of emotional meltdowns, others will take frustration in stride. A child's temperament is one reason for these differences in emotional reactivity. The other primary reason centers on the lessons you teach your child about how to develop emotional control, overcome frustration, and solve problems that come up in life.

If you are the parent of more than one child, you have probably noticed differences in your children's temperament, almost from birth. Some babies display the serenity of Gandhi, calmly and peacefully surveying the world. They lie in their cribs and occupy themselves looking at their mobiles while slurping on their fingers and toes. Nothing seems to trouble these kids. They easily accept smoochies from grandma, grandpa, and anyone else in the family.

Then there are kids who seem uninterested in faces and physical contact with family and friends. Occasionally, such children will have strong reactions to hugs, often yelling, screaming, and arching away. These children may seem independent, strong-willed, or "high-strung," showing anger over minor frustrations.

As babies grow, such differences in temperament continue. Some are highly active and quite loud, climbing on and over any object (including you) and screaming while they do so. They may take apart anything that isn't sealed tightly and work intensely to open anything that is. Any change in their daily schedule or frustration of their demands is met with tears or rage. At the other extreme, there are kids who are content to occupy themselves quietly while looking at picture books, watching television, or playing with toys. When it's time to stop play and go with Mom or Dad, it's no big deal. As parents, you have, I hope, fully realized that your parenting style did not cause these traits.

If you happen to be the parent of one child, you may also have noticed the differences between your child's temperament and that of other children. I hope you have recognized that you did not cause these differences either. The term *temperament* is typically used to refer to traits such as the child's activity level, degree of inquisitiveness, and the way he or she interacts with others and handles frustration. Is the child engaging or withdrawn? shy or outgoing? calm or easily upset? cheerful and optimistic or moody and complaining? Although there is considerable variability in people's energy level and emotional reactivity, one reality cannot be avoided: We all need to learn acceptable ways to express needs, tolerate temporary delays in satisfying our desires, solve interpersonal problems, and control our emotional reactions when we are disappointed or frightened.

As with the other lessons discussed, you will be your child's primary teacher, this time in the area of emotional and behavioral control.

In this lesson, I discuss strategies to help your child develop emotional control and inhibit impulsive behaviors (e.g., interrupting, intruding, demanding that needs be met immediately). Children, teens, and adults with attention-deficit/hyperactivity disorder (ADHD) commonly struggle with at least one of the following three types of emotional problems: outbursts of anger, excessive worry, and depressive reactions. The intensity of these reactions is far, far, greater than would be expected for the child's age group, often leading parents, teachers, and counselors to wonder if the child is really depressed; has an anxiety disorder, bipolar disorder, or a conduct disorder; or is a victim of abuse, rather than a child with ADHD. The following is an example.

Once I received a phone call from a highly concerned school social worker. One of my patients had become massively upset when he received his teacher rating for that afternoon. Apparently, he had not wanted to work on a particular school task and had resisted for a while. Although his teacher was able to coax him into working, he did not receive a smiley-face sticker for that time period. No big deal, right?

Well, when he saw the face without the smile, he freaked. He pounded his fist on the desk and pushed his papers and pencils off the desk, striking other students. He then proceeded to pound his head on the desk, saying, "I'm an idiot, I'm an idiot," followed by "I'm going to kill myself." He refused to do any more schoolwork and after much thrashing about, he was led to the social worker's office.

Once he got to the social worker's office, he continued to talk about wanting to kill himself. Like any trained professional, the social worker evaluated the risk for suicide. Did he have a plan?

Yep, he was going to go home, climb onto the roof of his house, and jump off. Was his mother going to be home so he could stop this? Nope, she was at work; only his older sister (a teenager) would be there. Clearly alarmed, the social worker contacted the mother and me. The social worker wondered if she needed to take the boy to the emergency room for crisis intervention. So far, this chain of events would make a lot of sense. Except for one detail: The child has ADHD.

WHAT DOES ADHD HAVE TO DO WITH A SUICIDE THREAT?

Long ago, when I first started treating kids diagnosed with ADHD, I might have done the same thing the social worker did. After all, there is a student in your office threatening a suicide, and the child has a plan that could certainly cause harm. That was before I realized that my patients would often have incredibly intense reactions to situations that didn't seem to merit it, such as threatening to kill themselves or run away because their parents wouldn't buy them a toy or take them somewhere. They would call themselves "stupid" or "an idiot," or say "I wish I were dead" because they couldn't figure out a math problem.

In contrast, if you have a child who has seemed depressed, irritable, moody, is withdrawing from friends, and doesn't seem interested in doing much of anything over the past week or two, and he or she starts to make comments such as "What's the point of living?" then there is cause for alarm, regardless of whether the child has ADHD. In this case, I'd encourage you to immediately contact your child's physician and arrange for an evaluation for depression and suicidal risk.

What I learned over the years is that most often, however, the causes of my patient's intense emotional reactions had more to do with the neurology of ADHD and adequacy of their diet, sleeping patterns, medication, educational plan, and communication and problem-solving abilities than with any type of trauma. This is different from what causes such reactions in children and teens who don't have ADHD.

The school example illustrates these differences. What if a child who didn't have ADHD had a meltdown over not getting a smiley face? Let's say this child talked about how he was going to kill himself. With such a child, I'd be very concerned about what was going on. I'd look to figure out what could possibly be triggering such a reaction in a child who typically did not show this type of behavior. Chances are that some pretty upsetting events had occurred or were occurring in that child's life.

However, if a child with ADHD starts expressing depressed or hostile thoughts because he or she didn't get a smiley-face sticker, my experience is that it is likely medication needs to be adjusted, diet and sleep habits examined, educational plan reviewed, or the parents' lesson plan for teaching problem-solving and anger-control skills needs to be revised. As I discuss in this lesson, most children with ADHD respond well to a combination of medication; instruction in problem-solving, social skills, and confidence-building techniques; and parental reinforcement of appropriate behavior when frustrated.

Although psychological factors are not at the root of most of the emotional or behavioral outbursts displayed by children with ADHD, it is important to realize that there are some children with ADHD who have experienced trauma, abuse, or neglect and that these children require psychological treatment. At my clinic, when a child continues to display intense anger, chronic depression, or debilitating anxiety despite a sustained period (6 months) of pharmacologic, nutritional, educational, and parental interventions, exploration of potential trauma, abuse, or neglect is often helpful.

With this in mind, let's think about what has happened when you have tried to help your child with ADHD calm down or cheer up when he or she is upset. I am certain you have attempted to have a rational conversation with your child who has ADHD when he or she was angry, frightened, or sad. What was that like? Were you able to discover the root of the intense emotional reaction and sanely address it? Highly unlikely! Remember that earlier in this book, I talked about the role of the frontal lobes of the brain. The frontal lobe has several jobs. One has to do with focused attention. However, another important role involves helping us think through situations that frustrate us and decide on an effective plan of action.

Most kids with ADHD have frontal lobes that are not sufficiently active. A smaller but significant percentage has overly active frontal lobes. As a result, when they need to pay attention or concentrate on school work, it is harder for them to do so. Similarly, when they are disappointed, frustrated, or scared, it is harder for them to use the thinking part of their brain to help control their emotional reactions and figure out another way to handle the situation. Until the rage or terror reaction subsides, there is really no way to talk rationally about the situation. Even more puzzling is the dramatic change that occurs in a child with ADHD within 10 minutes of the event if the parent, teacher, or counselor can stop feeding the emotional fire.

How Can I Not Feed My Kid's Emotional Fire?

Let's go back to the story of my maybe-suicidal patient. When I spoke to the school social worker, I asked if she was aware of what my patient would lose because of the teacher's rating. The social worker told me that the patient and his mother had made a deal for that day. The plan was this: If the child was able to get a smiley face for his effort and behavior for all four quarters of the day (they had divided the school day into four parts), he could go to his basketball game that night.

I encouraged the counselor to tell my patient that I would speak with his mother about their deal and see if there was any way he could make up for his mistake. However, the child needed to calm down (take some deep breaths, sip a little water, regroup, apologize to his teacher) and cooperate for the rest of the day. The counselor was asked to remind my patient that, as with other times when he had been disappointed and upset, he and his mom would figure out what to do to take care of the problem. The counselor also contacted his mother to make sure that an adult could be there after school.

When I spoke with the patient's mother, we reviewed several issues. One had to do with the all-or-nothing type of deal. These are real setups for meltdowns. Kids with ADHD are unlikely to be "perfect," so linking any type of reward to being perfect is unlikely to work. One goal behind reinforcement programs is to encourage effort, and my patient was certainly motivated to earn his reward. However, a secondary goal of any reinforcement program is to help a child learn how to control emotional reactions to frustration or disappointment. My patient was not so successful on that end, so my discussion with the mother centered on these two goals.

First, we looked at her child's effort for the day. Generally, it was quite good. After all, three smiley faces out of four is "not too shabby" (to quote Adam Sandler). But the child did "poop out" at the end and tried to avoid school work—not a good idea. We had to address that. In addition, his reaction to disappointment needed to improve. Here's what made sense to his mom. Because the child had resisted doing work at school, he needed to complete that assignment at home, plus some extra work, before Mom would consider letting him go to the game. Second, because he had done things that had frightened other people (kids in his class, the teacher, and the school social worker), he needed to do something to help them feel a little more relaxed.

At this point, my patient had to make a decision. He could refuse to do the work and not go to the game, or he could accept responsibility, perform corrective action (positive practice and positive punishment), and make amends. He chose to do the schoolwork (plus an extra assignment), and he decided to make a card for his teacher and for the social worker that included a joke from *Reader's Digest* (he cut it out) with some simple words to let them know he was sorry for worrying them but that he was OK and working on handling his anger better. He wasn't able to go out after school (because he was working on these tasks), but his mom let him go to the game because he took responsibility for his actions, performed corrective action (doing the avoided work plus an extra task), and took action to demonstrate sensitivity to the feelings of others.

The key elements in our plan were to continue to encourage the child's effort and emotional control and to help him realize that there are consequences when he tries to avoid work and when he loses his control. As I say throughout this book, it is important for parents to be clear about their lesson plan. Certainly, his mother could have stuck to her guns and held her line: "No four smiley faces, no basketball for you!" However, she is likely to have spent the rest of the day dealing with a determined, angry child who would pester her until it was too late to go to the game.

Of course, this mom could have kept piling on even more punishments for the child's behavior, which in turn would trigger another burst of emotional fire. I've seen kids with ADHD lose all privileges for a week within a few minutes because of their reactions to disappointment. However, at the end of the day, one of these kids is not likely to say, "I was wrong to give my teacher and parents a hard time. I know I need to do my work and try harder tomorrow." Nope. If Mom had held her hard line, adding punishments to the predictable outburst of begging, whining, tears, and rage, her son would have ended the night saying some version of "my mom's a jerk! I hate her!" If the child had lost privileges for the rest of the week, there would be even less motivation for him to try tomorrow. This can lead to a real downward spiral because a lack of effort at school will lead to fewer smiley faces, additional punishments, and so on.

TOOLS FOR EXTINGUISHING EMOTIONAL FIRES AND TEACHING CONTROL

Think about a time when your child had a meltdown. Ask yourself, "What did I want to teach?" "What was my lesson plan?" "How did my plan work?" As you are trying to reconstruct the scene, consider these keys for extinguishing emotional fires.

Key 1: Help the Child Find a Safe Place to Cool Off

What do you do when you're angry? Do you go and start talking to the person who ticked you off or to a passerby? As you have discovered, that is probably not a good idea. The reason? Anger is an emotional state intended to prepare us for a fight or to intimidate another person. During the time we are angry, the regions of the brain that are needed to solve a problem are not activated but suppressed. Consequently, the last thing that we should do when angry is talk with another person.

Step one in learning how to control anger is to remember not to speak to another person during that time. It will only lead to more trouble. Instead, your child needs to learn some ways to get the feeling to subside. Here are some ideas.

AT SCHOOL. A child can be given permission to see the school counselor, psychologist, or nurse; to take a walk with an aide; or go to a "chill-out area" in their school, if available. Children with ADHD who have a problem with anger control at school need to have such a plan in their Individualized Education Plan. That way, the teacher does not have to figure out what to say or do with a child who is obviously agitated, and the child will know that there is a way out of the situation without getting into more trouble. At the counselor's office, the child could work with clay or paint, listen to some music, sit in a comfy chair and grip a koosh (or stress) ball, or take a piece of paper and write (or type) everything he or she wanted to say (but didn't). These children can be shown how to use physical release to get the body to calm down a bit.

Showing and teaching kids the benefits of deep, slow breathing is my favorite stress-releasing activity. I share with kids what actually happens during angry moments. As soon as we see or hear something that triggers anger, we pretty much stop breathing. Heart rate speeds up, and oxygen flow to the brain drops off. Blood goes from the brain to the muscles, getting us ready to fight. I want my patients to learn that if they can start to breathe, then their anger will immediately drop off. So I tell them to begin taking one deep breath in . . . then another . . . then another. By the time they hit about five breaths, I tell them to begin asking themselves, What do I want? What can I do to make that happen? By the time they get to 10 breaths, they should be ready to start answering these questions. We practice that in my office, and I encourage them to do this at school as well.

Another strategy that some of my patients like is the Emotional Garbage Bag technique. Here's how it works. The Emotional Garbage Bag requires a paper bag, a piece of paper rolled into a megaphone, or some object that the child can yell into. The counselor can let the child know that when we get angry, there is a lot of "garbage" that builds up inside us and that we need to get rid of it before we can figure out what to do. The child is encouraged to put the bag over their mouth and say anything as loud as they want. If the child wants a target, the counselor can challenge the child to see if she or he can blow out the bottom of the bag with the force of their words. The bottom line is this: Before we try to figure out what to do, the child needs to reduce his or her anger. Either deep breathing in or expelling air out will reestablish air flow to the brain. I tell my patients that it is just not a good idea to talk to others when angry, so I practice what I preach in my sessions with them.

AT HOME. Cooling off by doing any nondestructive physical activity is a good idea (e.g., lifting weights, riding a stationary bike, hopping on a treadmill, playing an instrument, doing yoga, dancing, doing pushups or sit-ups, jumping on a trampoline). Listening to music, playing with clay or blocks, or using the Emotional Garbage Bag technique can also help. Because physically aggressive and destructive behaviors (pounding pillows, hitting a punching bag, kicking a ball) can establish a dangerous pattern for adult years, I do not encourage teaching children that engaging in aggressive behavior leads to a sense of physical release. I also find it useful for parents to practice deep, slow breathing exercises with their child. Once the child has reestablished his or her breathing, he or she can begin to answer the two frontal lobe questions ("What do you want?" "What can I do to make that happen?") and begin to solve the problem at hand.

Again, the key point to stress in your teaching is that we can talk about what to do when the child's anger subsides. I encourage parents to remind their children that they will be glad to talk with them once they have their breathing under control but that it doesn't make sense to talk to people when they are angry. If the child refuses to leave and insists on yelling at you, quietly remind him or her that the longer the yelling and screaming continues, the more he or she will need to do to make up for this decision. At that point, don't struggle with the child or try to force the child anywhere. However, when the child is finished, he or she will need to apologize to you (for not obeying you) and do whatever corrective action you consider appropriate.

Key 2: Identify the Child's Needs and Help Develop a Plan

When a child with ADHD is having an emotional outburst, identifying his or her need and developing a viable solution are crucial. As a parent, it may feel as though you are walking into a sea of emotional waves, but I encourage you to keep trying to bring the child to shore by encouraging her or him to remain quiet and continue breathing until he or she can identify the need and a way to make it happen. What did the child want or not want? Was it something that another child said or did? (*What did the child want?*) Was it a comment from the teacher? (*What did the child want?*). Was it a request to do work that the child does not know how to do? (*What did the child want?*) Was it the child's fear of your emotional reaction after school? In each case, the questions remain the same: "What did the child want? What can the child do to make that happen?" I tell my patients, "When you can answer these questions, your brain is back in the game. Until you can answer them, the only thing that can come from talking is more trouble."

Key 3: Help the Child Realize That If He or She Blew Up at Another Person, He or She Will Need to Apologize and Make Amends Before You Will Consider the Source of Frustration

After clarifying the nature of the need, you and your child can work on the problem at hand. As you do so, it is critical to realize that you are trying to help a child learn how to control emotional reactions and solve problems. If the child has yelled at or threatened another person, she or he will need to apologize and do something to make up. This doesn't have to be huge, but something needs to be done to reinforce the notion that if you mess up, you need to make up.

Key 4: Help the Child Learn Alternative Ways to Achieve a Personal Goal

Much as I hate to quote the Rolling Stones, a line from one of their songs has always made a lot of sense to me. I use it a lot (which must date me). The lyric is this: "You can't always get what you want, but if you try, sometimes you get what you need." In life, we don't always get what we want. But if we can fight the urge to rage or despair and get our frontal lobes into the game, typically we can figure out a way to get what we want or something just as satisfying. Let's play this out in a real-life situation.

A common problem that occurs at my office centers on where the family will eat lunch or dinner after an appointment with me. I have always preferred to locate my clinic on a street that has a variety of choices. In fact, I can easily boast that there is probably no clinic on the East Coast that has as many fast-food choices within two miles as mine. Name a food chain. Burger King? Got one. McDonald's? Got one. Wendy's? Yep. KFC? Yep. Subway? Yep. Want pizza? There's Pizza Hut, Domino's, and some local favorites (like Nick's, Tony's Nirchi's and OIP's) that make my taste buds sing. Need ice cream with that dinner? I've got Friendly's or Smarties (a local hangout). Give up yet?

Well, with all those choices, it's easy to generate frustration. Say you're thinking Pizza Hut but your child wants McDonald's. On your way to Dr. Monastra's office you make the mistake of bringing up the topic. An argument ensues. The child wants his burger, you want pizza. The kid begs, pleads, whines, sulks, and kicks the front seat. You hold on: "Pizza Hut or nothing," you say. The kid sulks and says, "I hate going to the doctor's and I'm not going in." You say, "If you don't go in, I'm going to _____" (the blank is provided for you to fill in your typical punishment or threat). The kid comes into the office obviously sulking.

After years as a psychologist, I've learned that if I react with a quiet, somber approach, the session will get off to a pretty lousy start. So I'd probably give the kid a great big greeting, toss a soft rubber ball in his direction, or see if he'll give me a hand on a Lego design in our waiting room's Lego Pit. I'd try any type of diversion that I could think of to get him moving (e.g., "Could you help me get a drink?" or "Could you help me figure out where I left the afternoon snack that I keep around for my patients?").

Once in my office (and away from the waiting-room audience), I'd mention in passing that it looked as though he was disappointed about something. Then I'd hear about the dinner tragedy. I'd check out how bad it had gotten (did he say anything horrific to his mom or dad?). I'd do that because I try to teach my patients that no matter how right you are, you need to apologize and make up for mean things that you say or do. If the child wanted to discuss this further, we'd go over ways to approach the parents. For example, when the child saw his parents, he could apologize and ask if there was anything he or she needed to do to make up for the actions that took place in the car. Then the child could ask if there was anything that could be done to convince them to go to McDonald's. If there was really nothing that could be done this time, then the child could try to obtain something else or discuss a way to get an agreement to eat at McDonald's the next time. The key element is to try to help the child learn how to solve problems by collaborating with (rather than bullying) others. I focus on this in the next lesson, and you'll get to play the role of parent-counselor.

Meltdowns in Other Public Places

This brings me to another common meltdown arena: the mall (or other outside shopping or recreational sites). Most parents try to prepare in advance for trips to these types of places. They are high-risk places for begging, whining, full-blown tantrums (when the child doesn't get his or her way), and general misery for parents. As a result, parents are advised to go over the ground rules with their children long before they leave the house and again before they get out of the car. If the child is going to be able to buy something, be clear about how much money he or she can spend and when it can be spent. If the child is not going to be able to buy anything but can earn a trip to a fast food restaurant, spell out what the child needs to do. It is important that you don't back yourself into a corner on this one. Here's an example of what I mean.

Let's say you're headed to the mall. You tell your children that you are going to get them sneakers. If they stay close to you, don't whine, and don't beg, then they can get a meal at Burger King. Sounds good, right? Hardly. From the minute you hit the mall, your child with ADHD is distracted by the wonder of it all and is begging to go into Video Game World, the arcade, the toy store, or any other place that seems neat. You say no again, and again, and again. Finally, you blow up and tell your child, "No Burger King!" The child goes ballistic. Big scene in the mall. All eyes are on you. You feel like an idiot. You are furious with your child and you exit the mall without sneakers. Don't feel bad if this has happened to you. It has happened to most (if not all) of us.

Think back on some of the earlier lessons. Remember the basic principle: If you want a child to learn, there needs to be a clear instruction given and a well-defined reason to learn. In addition, I talked about how the opportunity to earn what a child wants tends to promote improved effort. However, take-away types of punishment and removal of privileges really activates aggressive reactions in kids with ADHD. This is not to say that these kids should always get what they want. It just means they will learn much more from earning or failing to earn (their responsibility) rather than parental take-aways and loss of privileges (which translates to "My parents are jerks—it's their fault").

In the situation I just described, what is the instruction? "Stay close, don't whine, and don't beg." OK, that seems clear. Well, maybe not. How many times can the child wander, whine, or beg before the deal is off? Is it the first whine or the 30th? The first beg or the 50th? What it usually boils down to is how many times can the child not do what she or he was supposed to do before you blow up? You might think that it is highly understandable that the child loses Burger King after the tenth whine. But how did number 10 differ from number 9? Who was to know that the deal was 10 and out?

Here are a couple of ideas that may be useful. Let's say you are using a point system or chart at home. You could say that for every 5 or 10 minutes (depending on age) that the child stays within arm's reach, doesn't beg, and doesn't whine, the child earns a point. If it helps, he or she could even hold the watch or timer and keep track for you. The child needs a certain number of points to get to Burger King, but if the child doesn't earn BK, then he or she can use the points when you get home. However, as with other types of misbehavior, you will need to decide whether the child needs to make amends when you get home.

If you aren't using a point system, you could still use the 5- or 10-minute time approach and tell the child that he or she earns a quarter (or whatever seems reasonable) to use at Burger King (or another store) for each time period that the rules are followed. For every period, you can hand the child a penny or some type of token that could be exchanged for quarters at the desired location. If the child hasn't earned enough to buy a meal, then you will save it for the next trip to the mall. Again, if the child has a meltdown, it is pointless to try to reason with the child. It's probably best to leave the mall, regroup in the car (if possible) or try another time. Again, there are no "freebie" meltdowns. As we reviewed earlier, the child will need to apologize, practice listening to and obeying Mom or Dad (positive practice) and do something to make up for giving you such a hard time (positive punishment).

Remember, regardless of the intensity of your child's reaction, you are still the teacher. The child can yell and scream all she or he wants. If you have been requiring that the child follow the process we described in this book, there will need to be a lesson taught at home. Losing your control in the mall won't teach that. Repeating the process in which your child apologizes, practices, and makes it right will. You don't have to win the Battle of the Mall in front of bystanders. A calm reminder in the mall that the more the child misbehaves, the more he or she will need to do to make up is usually sufficient to get everyone moving out of the mall.

What About Medication to Help With Anger Control Problems?

There is a lot of debate about the use of medications in treating emotional problems in children. In some respects it parallels a broader issue among adults. After all, shouldn't people be able to control anger without resorting to drugs? Does this communicate that street drugs are OK? Won't it all lead to increased drug abuse among kids with ADHD? Finally, doesn't it mean that you are some type of defective parent if you even consider such a treatment?

A person's answers to these questions reveal his or level of knowledge when it comes to the kinds of emotional problems that people with different types of medical conditions can develop. Let's take diabetes, for example. If a person has a body that produces an insufficient amount of insulin, that person will have difficulty processing sugars. This condition is called *diabetes*. The American public is generally quite aware of this condition and considers it to be a "legitimate" medical condition. In fact, if a parent, grandparent, aunt, or uncle with diabetes started to seem extra tired, confused, grumpy, or outright hostile, family and friends might ask whether the person has eaten that day or checked blood sugar levels. With diabetic patients, the use of medication (and proper diet) serves several important roles. It helps stabilize blood sugar levels, which in turn improves attention, concentration, energy level, and mood. This doesn't mean that people with diabetes don't need to learn ways to control mood and solve personal problems. It just means that we need to attend to their medical care as part of the treatment.

Now let's consider a person with the medical condition called ADHD. Scientific evidence to date indicates that this condition is related to brain function, particularly in the level of activity in specific regions of the brain that are responsible for attention, concentration, mood regulation, behavioral control, and social judgment. The most commonly prescribed medications target those regions. When administered in a carefully titrated dose and in a context of adequate nutrition and sleep, these medications can help a child succeed in learning a number of skills, including the lessons described for controlling anger.

However, there are times when stimulant medications do not provide sufficient improvement in regions of the brain responsible for anger control. In those instances, several other types of medications may prove helpful. Antihypertensives (e.g., clonidine, Catapres) are the most commonly used type of medication to help with anger control issues. People with high blood pressure often use these medications to ensure that everyday stresses and frustrations do not significantly elevate blood pressure. Antihypertensives work by occupying brain receptors that are sensitive to adrenalin, a hormone that is released when we are experiencing frustrating or dangerous situations. When patients with ADHD use these medications, they are less likely to have aggressive outbursts over minimal frustrations. This type of medication can be used in combination with stimulants; however, monitoring of blood pressure is necessary to prevent excessive sedation. This type of medication has been approved by the Food and Drug Administration (FDA) for use with children with ADHD.

Antidepressant medications (e.g., Zoloft) and mood stabilizers (e.g., Abilify) are also occasionally used in the treatment of anger-control problems in children with ADHD. Although both types of medications seek to enhance the activity of neural pathways that promote calming, the side effect profile for antidepressants and mood stabilizers is significant. Children and teens using this type of medication can develop suicidal ideation, and withdrawal from these medications sometimes triggers hallucinatory experiences and marked worsening of mood. Consequently, they should be used with great caution and only after other, less risky interventions have been attempted. None of these medications have been approved by the FDA for use with children with ADHD.

Anticonvulsant medications (e.g., Depakote, Lamictal, Keppra) are sometimes used in the treatment of severe aggression in a child with ADHD. When used alone, they almost always cause increased inattention and impairment of concentration. Typically, they will be combined with stimulant medications to improve anger control and attention. However, as with antidepressants and mood stabilizers, this type of medication is typically only introduced after other interventions have proven ineffective. Again, caution is advised because none of the anticonvulsants have been approved by the FDA for use in patients with ADHD.

Depression, Phobias, and Anxiety Reactions

Up to this point, I have spent a lot of time discussing ways to help children with ADHD address feelings of anger and frustration. However, these children struggle with other types of emotional reactions too. Among the most alarming are the expressions of depression and the near-paralyzing levels of anxiety that can occur. I've watched kids burst out in tears, telling parents that they hated their lives and were going to commit suicide because they were being grounded for failing a course. I've heard stories about and have seen kids with ADHD who were nearly mute. These kids would go through extended periods of time appearing somber and unenthused about life, spending their time watching television or surfing the Internet for hours on end.

Certainly, the lack of emotional control during times of disappointment or frustration is not a trait unique to children and teens with ADHD. Let's face it, we all need to learn how to shake off the blues sometimes. However, certain kids with ADHD just don't seem thrilled about any part of life, whereas others react to the slightest disappointment as if it was the end of the world. To help kids with ADHD develop more resilience in dealing with disappointment and to reduce the degree of depression-like states, several strategies seem to be useful. I describe each in detail. Remember, although these strategies can be helpful, they are not likely to have a significant impact if your child is clinically depressed. As I mentioned in Lesson 3, consultation with a physician and consideration of a medication for depression are likely to be needed in those cases.

The first suggestion I give to kids with ADHD who are feeling depressed (and their parents) involves increasing the number of enjoyable activities that they do each day. Similar to eating "three squares a day," I encourage them to make sure they do three things they like every day. These little presents don't have to be huge, but just simple things. It could be making sure they get to watch a particular television show they like or getting the chance to snuggle and read a book with Mom or Dad. It could be a family game of Yahtzee or wearing a favorite sweater to school. It could be getting together with a friend or listening to music. It could be making sure they always have something they like for lunch (one of my favorites). Bottom line: Doing three pleasurable activities each day is a good "antidepressant" for anyone.

Another strategy to combat feelings of depression involves daily physical activity. Research evidence suggests that individuals can reduce symptoms of depression by engaging in activities such as walking, swimming, jogging, or biking for 20 to 30 minutes per day. I include research references on this topic in the Supplemental Resources. For kids, this translates to playing sports like baseball, soccer, football, swimming, wrestling, lacrosse, basketball, or tennis; practicing karate, gymnastics, or dance; or playing hide-and-seek, manhunt, or any other activity that involves getting the body into motion. Parents are advised to ensure that one of the requirements of daily life is that their child engages in such activities.

A third strategy ties into the concept of confidence. People who are depressed often have a low opinion about themselves. Here are some confidence builders to consider. It is important that a person feels that he or she looks good in the eyes of their parents. Even though it may seem like a no brainer, your child really needs to hear you say that you love him or her, and it is helpful for you to point out the times in the day that you are proud of them. Kids with ADHD often have a high rate of messing up. Their parents spend so much time correcting them that it is not surprising when one of my patients says to me, "My mom and dad don't like me much" or "I don't do anything right." If all you hear every day is some version of "don't do that" or "how many times do I have to tell you . . . ," it's hard to keep your head high. So look for the ways that your child shines. Kids with ADHD may have a hard time focusing on one thing but, wow, it's amazing what they do notice!

A related confidence builder has to do with the moral code that you are trying to teach your child. In his seminal text on self-esteem, Dr. Stanley Coopersmith pointed out that self-confidence is also related to the consistency between a person's lifestyle and his or her moral code. The more a person's actions were consistent with their moral code, the more self-respect or self-esteem they had. So instructing and encouraging your child to live by the foundations of your moral beliefs through your life stories and faith practices, as well as your social activities and choices of books, movies, television, and other media you use, will pay dividends when it comes to confidence.

Another booster shot involves helping your child become proficient at something that other kids of the same age respect or admire. Although it may be wonderful that your child develops awesome skills at the piano, this is not likely to help with confidence until late adolescence or college age. If your child loves playing the piano, riding horses, painting, and the like, that's great. However, try to make sure that the child is helped to "get good" at the kinds of activities that other kids in the neighborhood or school are involved in (playing various team sports, learning to play a band instrument, rollerblading, BMX racing, fishing, skiing, surfing, scouts, or joining a gymnastics, dance, swim, or karate club).

Confidence also comes from having at least one friend in your class. If your child routinely gets together with other kids in his or her class, great. If not, do what you what you can to learn the phone numbers of other kids in class and find ways to invite classmates over for informal gatherings or trips to a nearby park, fishing hole, lake, or other spot. Help your child find out what clubs, teams, or activities their classmates are in, and pave the way for your child to join up. For kids who live a distance from classmates, connecting with classmates at church groups, the YMCA or YWCA, a Boys & Girls Clubs of America, or interest groups (e.g., gymnastics, swimming, karate, BMX or microd racing clubs) can be helpful.

Don't be surprised if your fifth grader just wants to "veg out" on the couch and says doing anything other than watching TV or playing computer games is boring. That may be true at the moment. But just like you wouldn't be OK with him or her eating cookies all day ("because other foods are boring"), you can't be OK with your child retreating from activities that will help him or her grow in confidence. Doing none of these things is not an option. Even if you have to volunteer in class or at school activities so that you can find out the names and phone numbers of other kids (your child is not likely to ever do this on his or her own) or you have to add "participates in an activity with classmates" to the list of your child's daily responsibilities, do it! It will be well worth it.

Finally, we all feel better if we have a sense that we have some degree of control over our lives. Although you are the boss of your family, your child would get a boost if he or she has the sense of having some control over certain things. This could be what clothes to wear to school, the color of his or her bedroom walls, or the choice of meals one day per week. It could be the choice of one family activity per month. It's your call. Have some fun with this.

My Child Is Too Terrified to Do Anything With Other Kids. What Can I Do?

Anxiety and phobic reactions are common among my patients. As with anger control issues, antihypertensive medications and antidepressants are the primary types of medications that could be considered, if you are comfortable with the use of medicines. Between the two types, antihypertensives have fewer side effects, work more immediately, and are easier to discontinue. Guanfacine (brand name: Tenex) has been approved by the FDA for use in children. It is available in a pill form that lasts about 6 hours or a sustained release form (Intuniv) that can last up to 12 hours. None of the antidepressant medications (e.g., Paxil, Celexa) have been approved by the FDA for use in children, so I'd encourage you to consider other types of interventions first. At our clinic, we have found antihypertensives to be well tolerated and useful when combined with low doses of Adderall-XR or Vyvanse to boost attention. However, my experience has been that unless guanfacine or Intuniv are used in combination with a stimulant medication, they are often too sedating.

Isn't There Something I Can Do Besides Give My Child Medication?

In addition to medications, there are several strategies that parents can use to reduce fears. Each of these strategies is founded on the following well-established principle: If we face what we fear and experience a sense of calmness (or a relaxed state) while we are in the fear-evoking situation, then our fears begin to subside." I'll start with a simple example and expand from there.

I knew a child who was afraid to go outside because she had been told (by a friend) that if she touched a particular type of bug, she would turn into that bug. Things got so bad that the child began avoiding going outside and insisted on being carried everywhere. So what could her parents do? Well, most of us would start off by trying to convince the child that there was nothing to worry about. That approach will go nowhere fast. I learned a long time ago that you cannot reason away fears. It eventually boils down to a person's decision to enter into the "fear zone" and take a chance that he or she will survive. Now, the word of an expert (like a parent) might help, but the odds are high that some type of direct exposure will be needed. So I talked with the child about the truth (i.e., touching a slug would not turn you into one) and went outside and just looked at some for a while. However, the turning point came when I showed the child that touching was safe (by me touching one), and we both saw that I survived.

This example of the bug phobia is just one example of the kinds of fears kids have. Some are afraid to go alone into parts of the house or apartment. In those cases, I often encourage parents to play a kind of hide-and-seek game in which the parents hides boxes in different parts of the house. Some will contain little gifts (e.g., a snack, a dime, or a ticket for game time with Mom or Dad). Other boxes will contain words of encouragement (e.g., "I can't believe you were brave enough to go under the bed. I'm proud of you!"). Still others might contain something that the child is afraid of (e.g., a jar with a spider in it). As the child searches for little prizes, the child overcomes the fears.

Another common fear involves sleeping alone at night. Although it may seem easier to just give in to our child's desire, once children get into the habit of sleeping with their parents, they strenuously resist sleeping alone. In addition to the obvious limitation on parental intimacy, when a child is allowed to sleep with Mom and Dad, it contributes to the avoidance of facing and mastering one of the earliest childhood fears: "I can be OK even when I am sleeping without a parent in the room." Because confidence comes from facing fears, your permission to allow a child to sleep with you interferes with developing the confidence that comes from overcoming this fear.

When kids have a fear of sleeping alone, I often use the following approach. We start out by establishing a specific time for going to the child's bedroom each night. In addition, we make sure that the child does not snack on high-energy foods (e.g., cookies, chocolate, caffeinated beverages) and discontinue use of electronic screens (TVs, video games, computer games, etc.) at least 1.5 hours before bedtime. Until the child is consistently sleeping alone, I want to make sure she or he is not surfing a sugar or adrenalin high while trying to get to sleep.

The next step involves moving a chair for the parent into the child's room. This chair needs to be comfortable enough so the parent can sit a while and read the paper or a book (with the assistance of one of those miniature book lights), as the child falls asleep. With the lights on in the room, the parent can read to the child, either while sitting on the child's bed or in the parent chair. However, after reading, the lights need to be dimmed and the child is to stay in bed. The parent informs the child that she or he will stay in the room and watch over the child. A mother might let her child know that she'll also be checking in on Daddy during the night. There is minimal conversation after this point. As with any skill, it is often helpful for the parent to give the child a reason for learning to face this fear. This could be the opportunity to do some "big boy" or "big girl" activity the next day, the chance to earn money toward a prize at the end of the week, or being able to have a favorite breakfast or lunch item the next day. Letting the child know that he or she will "feel so proud when (he or she) can sleep alone" in the bed may also help.

After the child demonstrates that she or he can fall asleep within 15 minutes with the parent in the room, the parent chair is moved to the doorway. The process remains the same. There is reading time with the child and then quiet time. The parent remains in the doorway in the chair until the child demonstrates that she or he can fall asleep within 15 minutes on a consistent basis. At this point, the parent can then begin to go outside the child's room after reading. The parent typically will need to be on the same floor of the house until the child falls asleep.

As with any plan, there can be problems with this one. Your child may refuse to stay in bed and may insist on sitting on your lap. As with any refusal, I encourage you to let the child know that the longer the child resists and the more work the child causes for you, the more he or she will need to do for you the next day before playtime. Another typical problem occurs if the child wakes up in the middle of the night and calls out for you. Much as you'd rather stay in bed, I encourage you to tuck your child in and remain in your "parent chair" until the child falls asleep.

Even though this may seem like a lot of work, facing the fear of the dark at bedtime contributes to a child's sense of power and confidence. Although there are children's books and videos that can help a bit, in the end, it will boil down to your child's decision to face these fears. It is essential for the development of confidence that your child (and you) succeed at this task.

Again, as with the other emotional control problems, some parents will use medications to help in this process. When the strategies we discussed are insufficient, some parents use the antihypertensives we discussed in this lesson and elsewhere in the book. Some parents may also try melatonin supplements for a short time. If the issue is primarily fear (rather than a sleep disorder), melatonin supplements or antihypertensives can be helpful.

With children who seem generally anxious, I also use a bravery game to build confidence. Again, awarding points, privileges, or activities for facing fears is recommended. In the bravery game, parents work with their child to develop a list of activities and things that the child fears (I encourage parents to also develop their version of this list to make the bravery game more fun). After the list is developed, parents can teach their child about the calming effect of controlled breathing, and the parents can then help their child face one fear per day or week. When I teach a child (or anyone) about controlling anxiety by breathing, the person is initially doubtful until I demonstrate. Here's a lesson that you might find useful.

I begin the lesson by telling kids one important truth: "You can't feel anxiety if your body has plenty of oxygen (air)." I continue with some version of

> When we are in a situation that scares us, the first thing that happens is that we stop breathing (I show them what being scared looks like and how we just stop and freeze). As soon as we stop breathing, our heart goes into overdrive. It starts beating faster and faster, trying to get the little bit of oxygen to all the body parts that it can. We feel that as anxiety, fear, or worry. The more worry we feel, the less we breathe. This keeps our heart going faster and faster until we feel dizzy and might even pass out. We try to tell ourselves to calm down, but that doesn't work. Usually, the worry only fades when we run away (or avoid) the situation. That works fine for the time being, but it doesn't help us get over our fears.
>
> So if you want to get over your fear, the most important thing you need to learn is to feed your body some oxygen (or air) as soon as you start to worry. Once you start giving your body some nice, deep, drinks of air, you're on the way to feeling great again. You see, as soon as your body starts to get some air, your heart doesn't have to work so hard. It can start to slow down. As you feel your heart slow down, you'll feel less worried, and pretty soon, you're OK. You just need to remember that the heart might need you to give it at least 15 to 20 slow, deep nose-fills before it has enough air for your body.

I practice this a bit with the child. Try this with your kid (or yourself). You'll be amazed.

HOMEWORK

In this lesson, I reviewed ways to help your child with such common emotional problems as outbursts of anger, depressed mood, fears, and anxiety. If your child is struggling with any of these problems, now is a good time for you to sit back and think about your plan to teach your child ways to control these emotional states. You may decide to contact your doctor to discuss medication as part of the plan. That is absolutely fine. There is no extra credit given for parenting without medicine, especially if your child does not seem to be making any progress without it. Chronic anger, depression, and anxiety do not build character; they tear it down. Regardless of your decision to use medication or not, my hope is that you will decide on a "lesson plan" to begin to develop your children's confidence and ability to use certain psychological strategies to control mood and improve their success in handling the problems they'll face in daily life. These are among the most important lessons that you will teach your children.

One final thought: In this lesson, we have discussed a number of strategies to help your child overcome feelings of intense anger and depression and crippling anxiety. However, if your child is expressing anger and depression by making statements such as "I wish I was dead" or "I'm going to kill myself," you need to contact your child's doctor or therapist so that they can evaluate the risk of harm to your child or others. Although kids with ADHD may simply make a suicidal or homicidal statement because they can't figure out a better way to express themselves, it is better to seek help immediately rather than wait.

LESSON 9

YELLING RARELY SOLVES ANYTHING

I often tell parents that the first lesson they teach their children is that Mom and Dad will love and care for them. If the child will accept hugs, kisses, and close physical contact during infancy and early childhood, many "I love yous" are smothered on the child without much thought. If babies smile, the world opens up to them. If babies need a hug, some food, a diaper change, something outside of their grasp, or some playtime, crying will usually get the desired response from a caring parent. However, once children reach an age when crying is no longer an acceptable way to get what they want (somewhere around age 2 years), problems begin. We not-so-jokingly refer to this time period as the *terrible twos*. After a child learns to speak, crying to get something typically irritates parents. Whining, begging, and throwing tantrums aren't appreciated either. Outright defiance of a parent's rules really pushes buttons.

As we go through the years and our children become teens and young adults, children must learn new ways to get what they want. At first, they'll use variations of what worked when they were babies. They'll cry, whine, yell, and beg. They'll throw tantrums. They'll regress to the age of 3 or so and keep asking, "Why?" "Why do I have to go to bed now?" "Why do I have to do homework?"

"Why can't I buy a new video game?" "Why can't I have my own phone, iPad, etc.?" "Why do I have to eat breakfast?" Or they'll beg, "Pleeeeeese mommy . . . pleeeese?" On and on and on. Any time you are at the grocery store, or the local burger place, or the mall, it won't take too long before you see a child much older than 3 still using these "baby" strategies to get what he or she wants (I hope it won't be your kid, but hey, it just might be). At some point, we come to recognize that there is another critical lesson our children need to learn: How to get what they want while respecting the needs and concerns of other human beings.

From the time you and your child wake up in the morning, you are immersed in the process of solving problems. You need to immediately orchestrate the tasks of waking, washing, feeding, and dressing not only for yourself but also for your children. Later, you and your children will need to figure out who is going to cook, clean, and pick up clothes, toys, and junk. You and the kids will be involved in negotiating playtime, television time, computer time, homework, chores, bedtime, meals, and everything else that make up your daily activities. You will decide on purchases, travel to a friend's house, the mall, and so on. These are just a few of the many decisions that you and your children will make on a daily basis. How you choose to handle these decisions determines whether you will end up with a teen who is acting like a "baby" or one who has learned how to solve problems in a mature way. Although most examples in this lesson focus on teens, the lesson can, and ideally should, be used with younger children too, adapted to their level.

TEACHING PROBLEM-SOLVING SKILLS

Let's take a couple of minutes to think about some common ingredients in a typical parent–child argument. Typically, problems occur if there is a conflict of needs or if one person wants something that the other person doesn't want or is afraid to give. If a parent wants a child to do something and the child says "OK," then there's no issue. If a child wants something and a parent says "OK," "Sure," or "No problem," no sweat. The child smiles, is glad to have gotten what she or he wanted, and all is well. But what happens if a parent says no? Or if the child ignores, defies, or argues with a parent's request or decision?

Behind most (if not all) "no's" is some kind of fear, worry, or competing need. Our kid asks to stay up later. We are concerned that the child will be a bear in the morning, and so we say no. Our 14-year-old wants to go to the mall with some friends. We fear the teen may be abducted, harmed, or encounter some other dangerous situation, and so we say no. You're just getting in the door after work. You no sooner get inside than your kid wants to know if you will take her to the store. Chances are, you will immediately feel a kind of "digging in," a sort of resistance. You just got home and now you are being asked to go out. The child has a need for something (a toy, a video, or something for a school project). You have a need for something else (rest, food, etc.).

Now, you have every right to *just say no*. That's OK. Let's face it, not everything is up for discussion. I'd be the last one to say we have to talk about our fears or needs to get our 4-year-old to eat some veggies. However, I'd like you to begin to realize that some of the day-to-day "conflicts" with your child can become teaching moments.

Children need to learn that when they want something and another person says no, chances are good that the other person is concerned about something or has competing needs. Instead of whining, begging, yelling, or throwing a tantrum, kids need to learn to discover what the other person fears or wants to resolve the conflict. Solving problems with another person means that you try to get what you want while paying attention to the concerns and needs of the other person. That is the heart of the matter. Let's go over some of the more important steps in teaching your child.

STEP 1: LEARNING TO EXPRESS NEEDS IN A RESPECTFUL WAY

How would you like your child to ask for something? "Hey mom, I need to go to. . . ." "Dad, drive me to Billy's!" "Dad, you've got to take me to school in 10 minutes." "Mom, give me $10 for the movies!" Most of us don't like being bossed around by our kids. I can't imagine you do, either. So Step 1 in problem solving is for your child to learn what you consider a respectful way to ask for something.

How would you like your child to make requests? Is "May I," "Please," "Is it OK if," or "If it's not a problem for you Dad, could you . . . " what you'd like to hear? If so, then you need to teach your child that skill. As with all the other lessons I talk about in this book, learning how to make a request or begin a discussion is important. Your child may want something, but so do you. You probably want respect and maybe a bit of appreciation. There is nothing wrong (and a lot right) about making sure that your child addresses your need to be respected or appreciated when he or she wants something. Kids with ADHD (like other kids) need to learn how to be sensitive to the needs and feelings of others. You need to be your child's teacher.

What If My Kid Ignores My Requests to Ask for Things in a Respectful Way?

Remember when I discussed Time Stands Still in Lesson 7? If your child ignores your requests to be spoken to respectfully, let her or him know that you aren't going to consider any requests until the child apologizes, does something to make amends, and speaks to you respectfully. Kids with ADHD can be intense and demanding. However, they can also learn that if they are disrespectful, they are postponing getting what they want. They can learn that disrespect leads to a need for an apology, making up, and then starting all over again.

STEP 2: UNDERSTANDING THE CONCERNS AND NEEDS OF OTHERS

OK. Let's say your child has asked for something in a way that is respectful. Great! Now what? Well, now is the part that gets personal. If this is one of those times that you'd like to do a bit of teaching, you'll need to ask yourself a couple of questions.

> Question 1: "Am I thinking about saying no because I'm concerned about something?" (Here you are trying to figure out if the "no" is because of some type of worry or fear.)
>
> Question 2: "Am I thinking about saying no because I want something from my child?" (Here you are trying to figure out if a "no" is because of some kind of need that you have.)

Check yourself out. Let's play out a couple of situations.

Your 14-year-old daughter is asking to go to the movies with friends. You are feeling the urge to say no (I sometimes describe this as feeling "no-aliscious"). You say, "I'm not sure about that." Instead of begging or whining, your daughter learns to ask a simple question. She asks, "What are you worried about, Mom?" After you pick yourself up from the floor, you ask yourself, "OK, what am I worried will happen if I say yes?" Here are some possible concerns:

- My child won't be safe. She'll get hurt or abducted.
- My child will hang out in a place where kids smoke or use drugs.
- My child will pick up some bad habits by watching a certain movie.
- My child won't get her homework done.
- My child will stay up too late and not get up for church the next day.

This list is by no means exhaustive, but it's a starting point. The first question that needs to be asked and answered if you're thinking "no" because of worry is this: "What am I concerned will happen?" For example, maybe you are thinking "no" because you're concerned your child will be hurt or abducted. If that's the case, then that's where you and your child start the problem solving. The problem for your child has now become the following: "How can I go to the movie and respect Mom's worry that I might get hurt or abducted?"

At this point, you can pull out a piece of paper and write down possible ways to address your safety concerns and still allow your child to go to the movies. What are some options? You and your child can sit down and take turns generating possible solutions. If your child starts to insult you (e.g., says you are being stupid), then just like before, she will need to regroup, apologize, and, if needed, do something to make up. Your child needs to learn that insulting another person is not a good problem-solving strategy. As long as the child is being respectful, you can proceed to list possible solutions. Here are several possibilities:

1. There should be at least four kids going to the movies. Mom drops me off and picks me up in the lobby of the theater.
2. Sally and I take a bus to the theater, and I bring my cell phone in case of trouble.
3. Mom drops off Sally and me and picks us up in the lobby of the theater.
4. Mom watches the movie with me and my friends.
5. My 18-year-old brother goes with us.
6. Mom and Dad go to one movie; my friends and I go to another movie at the same theater. We go into the theater together and leave together.

The problem-solving phase requires that your child realize she needs to respect your concerns while attempting to get what she wants. If you are not comfortable with Sally and your daughter taking the bus, then that option is out. The only way your daughter gets to go is if she agrees to an option that addresses your concerns. You could decide that Options 1, 4, 5, and 6 are OK with you. Your daughter could decide which of those choices she likes. The essential lesson is this: In solving life's problems, a person needs to address the concerns of parents, friends, teachers, coworkers, employers, spouse, and/or partner.

Let's say the worry is that if your daughter goes to the movie, she will not complete her homework. If that's the case, then the problem for our child to solve is, "How can I go to the movie and also address Dad's concern that I won't do my homework?" Options to consider might include the following:

1. I do all my homework before going to the movie.
2. I do half my homework before the movie and complete the other half on Sunday before I get to watch television or do anything fun.
3. I promise to do my homework sometime before the weekend is over.

Let's say that you're only OK with Option 1 because Sunday is a day you spend at church or typically do something else as a family. Then your daughter would need to agree to that or come up with another solution that will address your concern that homework won't get completed.

What If I'm Not Afraid or Concerned? What If I Just Don't Feel Like Saying Yes?

Not all requests meet with a parental no because of worry. Sometimes, the parent is feeling fatigued, burdened, or has some other need. If that is the case, your child needs to learn to ask Question 2: "Dad, is there anything I can do for you so you'll let me do (whatever), or so that you'll do (whatever) for me?" This question is designed to help your child figure out what you need so that you will say yes. If fear or concern is not part of the reason that you are saying no to a request, then chances are you have a need that should be addressed. Let's go back to the movie request.

What if the reason you are saying no to the movie request is because you feel tired; you feel like a slave to your kids; you feel as though you are the only person who does anything. So you ask yourself, "What do I need?" or "What does my child need to do so I'd be OK with taking her to the movies?" Instead of saying "No, I'm too tired," you could tell her your needs, like this:

> I could really use a break before dinner. I wanted to unwind and watch a program I recorded. I was going to try to watch it after dinner, but if you'll help me prepare the meal, I'll take you and Sally to the movie. Here's what I want you to do. I'd like you to make the spaghetti and heat the sauce. First, I want you to fill this large pot with water (up to here) and wait for it to boil. Once it starts to boil, let me know.

After the water boils and your daughter comes to you, you continue your instructions:

> OK, the next part of your job is to put a box of spaghetti in the pot and set the timer for 10 minutes. I also want you to heat the sauce that I've put in this pot on the stove. I don't want you to leave the kitchen because you have to stir the pots and make sure the spaghetti doesn't stick and the sauce doesn't burn. Any questions? OK, then, we have a deal. You take care of dinner prep while I watch my program, and I'll take you to the movie after you clean up the dishes.

In this situation, the daughter was able to take care of her need by paying attention to her mom's need for some rest and relaxation. A pretty common parental need is for some help with the family's work. However, there is another need most parents have: They need to feel loved, wanted, or appreciated by their child.

Let me tell you a brief story. I once worked with a family who was struggling with their teenager's desire to spend every waking moment with his friends. The parents tried to do the best they could to get him to his friends' homes. However, one particular weekend, the father said no to his son, telling him he couldn't go out with his friends that weekend. The boy went nuts. He'd done everything that he was supposed to do, hadn't gotten into any trouble at school, so "Why, why, why?!!!" couldn't he go out? However, the teen tried to solve the problem like a baby, failing to realize that his dad must have wanted or was concerned about something to have said no. After the dust settled, the teen learned that the simple reason his father wanted him home was that his dad missed spending time with him. But his dad never said that, and the boy never asked. The result was a huge fight.

In the end, his father realized that he had to accept his son's need to be with his friends. His son learned that he had to become aware of his dad's needs too. In this case, the father and son decided to plan some time for skiing together (with mutual family friends) so that they could spend time going on some runs together and the son could continue to develop the friendships that were so important to him.

The sense of loss that a parent feels over the limited time spent with a child (particularly during the teenage years) is common, but it is not just a problem for the parent. Although teenagers will spend the vast majority of their time talking, texting, on Facebook, Tweeting, visiting, and traveling with their friends, spending some time with parents remains important for the child's development during adolescence. Without any social or recreational contact with parents during adolescence, the parent–teen relationship deteriorates and conflict over typical teenage requests commonly escalates. In addition, those parent–teen moments on a lake, outside gazing at the stars, hiking, stacking firewood, fishing, taking a round of golf, playing a driveway game of PIG on the basketball court, swimming in the pond, playing video games, getting sprayed by a hose or a just-sprung fire hydrant, or munching on a late night pizza or grabbing an ice cream cone convey love and teach lessons that your child can't get from friends.

HOMEWORK

The basics of solving problems between two people involve recognizing and respecting each person's needs and concerns. This is an important lesson for anyone to learn and apply. As is true with any lesson I discuss in this book, learning takes practice. Before you begin teaching this new skill, let your child know that you want to teach him or her another way to talk about problems. Tell the child your version of the story about how babies get what they want by crying, whining, and yelling, but as we grow up, we all have to learn a more grown-up, mature way. Then sit down with him or her and use your variation of the Problem Worksheet that follows.

Problem Worksheet

What does your child want? _____

What's making you want to say no?

Is it a need? Ask yourself, "What do I want?" List it below.

_____

_____

Is it a fear or concern? Ask yourself, "What am I afraid of?" List it below.

_____

_____

Solving this problem means that you and your child will need to take care of what the child needs, as well as your needs and concerns.

So what ideas do you and your child have that could solve this problem?

1. _____

2. _____

3. _____

4. _____

5. _____

6. _____

After you list about six ideas, stop and cross out any that you (or your child) are not comfortable with, and select a solution from what remains. If you've crossed everything out, take a little time off (half an hour or so) and try again.

© Vincent J. Monastra, PhD

NOW THAT YOU HAVE THEIR ATTENTION, WHAT DO YOU REALLY WANT THEM TO LEARN?

So far, we've covered a lot of information about attention-deficit/ hyperactivity disorder (ADHD) and some of the more common problems that kids with this condition have to face and solve. However, during the past decade, a very different type of question started to creep into my thinking. Then one day, a simple truth hit me: I had spent my career trying to help kids pay attention, without ever asking their parents, "What do you think is really worth paying attention to?" That led to a series of great conversations and the foundation for this lesson.

What I learned is that beyond picking up, not fighting with their siblings, getting their homework done, and graduating from high school (and typically college), many parents were concerned that their children were not being taught the kinds of values that most of us admire in our heroes and wish we could instill in our children, if only we had the time. We watch programs on television, and every so often we'll hear an inspirational story about a child who distributes sandwiches to homeless people or a little girl who creates a lemonade stand that becomes a lightning rod for funding medical research (you might want to read the story about Alex's Lemonade Stand: www.alexslemonade.org). The parents that

I spoke to wanted their children to become people with real conviction to do the right thing. They just hadn't really thought about how to do it.

So I started asking parents some questions about the values they'd like to teach. I wasn't really surprised at the top dozen. Here's the short list (in no particular order). Parents wanted their children to learn

- to be generous, compassionate, hardworking and kind;
- to be thoughtful, honest, grateful, and patient;
- to be hopeful, responsible, trustworthy, have faith in God;
- to follow their family's moral and spiritual values; and
- to have the conviction to stand up for what was right.

Above all, parents simply said that they wanted their child to be happy. Their belief was that if they could help their child develop these kinds of traits, then their son or daughter would have a better chance at achieving happiness. They were concerned that something was getting lost in all the focus placed on helping kids with ADHD sit still and pay attention. They felt like they weren't really taking the time to talk to their kids about what really mattered and that their child was losing the sense that they were good or worthwhile because they were constantly being corrected for doing things wrong.

As I was talking with these parents, I started thinking about the research of Dr. Martin Seligman at the University of Pennsylvania. For decades, psychologists like Dr. Seligman have been trying to get a better understanding about the sources of happiness. In the book *Flourish: A Visionary New Understanding of Happiness and Well-Being* (2011), he provides a pretty comprehensive picture of what contributes to a state of happiness and well-being.

No surprise, Dr. Seligman found that a state of happiness and well-being certainly ties into how often life gives you something you like. Someone smiles at you, acts interested in what you are saying, tells you they like you or gives you a hug—all those experiences generate a positive feeling that we'd call "happiness." Or you find out that you earned a bonus at work, or your child made the Honor Roll, or you enjoyed a day at the park with your family and the kids somehow magically all got along—and you feel "happy." But happiness is not limited to moments when things go the way that we like. If we simply waited around for life to go our way, most of us would be waiting a long time.

What most parents realize is that they need to teach their children other skills to help them develop that sense of feeling "well" or "happy." That's what they were sharing with me when we spoke at my clinic. And that's what Dr. Seligman found in his research. Developing traits such as optimism, resilience, inquisitiveness, and self-confidence plays a big part in a person's feeling happy. In this lesson, we'll talk about how to develop some of these traits.

So what do you *really* want your child to learn? Let's start by taking a look at the list of traits that we developed after talking with parents who brought their children to our clinic. Here's the list in checklist form. Take a few minutes and check off what you'd like to teach your child.

As you did when you completed the list "What I Want My Child to Learn," select two or three values that you'd like to begin to teach your children. With my 8-year-old boys, the biggies have been helping them become more compassionate, generous, and kind. So here's one example of how we are beginning to teach compassion and generosity.

At Christmastime, my sons were all pumped up about getting every Star Wars Lego kit imaginable. Every morning, they'd come

---

Parent Values Checklist

I'd like my child to become more

1. ___ Generous	11. ___ Grateful
2. ___ Compassionate	12. ___ Resilient
3. ___ Hardworking	13. ___ Determined
4. ___ Kind	14. ___ Creative
5. ___ Thoughtful	15. ___ Loyal
6. ___ Honest	16. ___ Cheerful
7. ___ Patient	17. ___ Friendly
8. ___ Hopeful	18. ___ Inquisitive
9. ___ Trustworthy	19. ___ Confident
10. ___ Connected with God	20. ___ Responsible
(or our family's moral and	
spiritual values)	

© Vincent J. Monastra, PhD

---

to the breakfast table armed with the latest advertisement from Toys"R"Us or Target and go on and on about how they needed to get the X-Wing or Tie Fighter. I woke up to the reality that I needed to begin to teach them about compassion and generosity when they came in determined to get a Death Star for Christmas.

Now for those of you who have no idea what a Lego re-creation of the Death Star costs, I'll give you a hint. You probably could pay your utility bill for a month for what it costs at this time ($399). You also could sponsor a starving child in Africa, Asia, Central America, or some other impoverished region of the world for a year. I decided to take this moment to teach my sons something pretty important: the values of compassion and generosity.

Because we had recently gone to one of their friends' birthday parties, I said some version of "I think the Death Star looks pretty cool, but I thought we were celebrating Jesus' birthday at Christmas. Remember when we went to your friend Joshua's party, we tried to figure out what he would like, right?" Of course my boys nodded. I continued, "Joshua seemed to like what we picked out, and he even gave you a present too, didn't he?" More nods, but I could see that "Where's Dad going with this?" look on their faces. "OK," I said, "So let's think about what Jesus told us that He liked. I know that He told us to be kind, love each other, and give to the poor." My boys remembered that and again nodded. So I said, "For $399 we could buy the Death Star or we could feed a child in Africa for a year. Which do you think would make Jesus happier?" Without blinking, my boys said, "Feed a child in Africa," which is what we did and continue to do to this day.

Now my sons did receive presents at Christmastime, but the Death Star wasn't one of them. And no, we didn't make up for the missing Death Star by purchasing something just as expensive. We did buy them several gifts, and they were thrilled to get to play with their toys. And they also got one other gift. Every couple of months, they get a letter from their new Kenyan friend, Fatuma, who thanks them for their generosity and gives them a little bit of an idea of what it's like to grow up in Africa.

Although this example reflects my family's Christian beliefs, compassion is a value shared by people with a wide range of perspectives on religion. Taking the time to reach out and share our time, talents, and resources is not just a Christian trait, a Jewish trait, a Muslim trait, or limited to kind people who volunteer through the Red Cross, United Way, or other agencies. It feels good for everyone and can help create a much safer, loving, and fun world. So if you happen to be a member of a religious organization, find out how your child can participate in their outreach efforts. If you are not a member of such a community, use a website such as Charity Navigator with your kids to learn ways to show compassion. Your child might really develop some great values. Here are a few ideas:

- Donate animals to people in impoverished areas.
- Support a business in a developing part of the world with a microloan.
- Volunteer or give money to disaster relief efforts.
- Help elderly neighbors with lawn care, snow removal, home repair, and other chores.
- Explore ways to provide housing through Habitat for Humanity.
- Write to your senator or representative to advocate for legislation to help a cause that is important to you.
- Volunteer at an animal shelter, food bank, or fundraiser for a community need.

Bottom line, Christmas and the other winter holiday celebrations are a great time to begin to teach generosity and kindness. Whether your family celebrates Christmas, Hanukkah, Kwanzaa, or the Sweet Festival that comes at the conclusion of Ramadan, the common themes of each of these festivals encourage thanksgiving, acts of charity, and giving gifts to those we love.

BUT MY KIDS WILL THROW A FIT IF WE MAKE THEM GIVE UP THEIR HOLIDAY GIFTS!

If you're thinking that, you're not alone. A lot of us have spent way too much money on stuff that we know isn't great for our kids. But we do it so they won't be disappointed or, maybe more to the point, so they won't get mad or whine. One of the classic examples of this type of guilt or "keep the kids quiet" spending comes all wrapped up at the holidays in little packages containing video games and other types of electronic entertainment devices. Now I really don't believe that too many of us would say, "I think it's good for my kid to sit around involved in an endless battle experience." But the truth is, our kids are quiet for hours and hours and hours as they work their way through the action on Halo, Call of Duty, Star Wars, Mario Brothers, or whatever other high-action game they love. Besides, if we didn't buy them these presents, wouldn't they get mad at us? Well, they probably would. But are we buying a good kind of quiet?

So now that you're taking a few minutes to think about what you want to teach your kids, I want to ask you one question: Why are you letting your kids play these games for hours on end? Be honest. Is it because "it keeps them quiet"? That much is probably true. I've never found a babysitter who could keep kids as engaged as an X-Box. Is it because "if my kid doesn't play these games, he won't have friends"? If you're thinking that, then you might be surprised to learn that the opposite is actually true. The tendency is for intense gamers to have relatively few friends outside of the cyberworld. The pattern of social isolation associated with playing electronic games on the Internet or on the various game boxes can continue into adulthood unless a parent intervenes. Is it because "they don't want to do anything else, and I'm too tired to fight"? If that's the case, then I surely understand, but we've got to find a way to boost your energy. You see, people can debate all they want about whether playing video games causes kids to become violent, but I think that misses the point. The truth is that these games are highly enjoyable for kids but don't typically teach them the values we want them to learn, and they can be highly addictive.

HOW ARE VIDEO GAMES ADDICTIVE?

Yep, video games are addictive. The truth is that just like the old Lays potato chip commercial, "no one can eat just one." Kids don't play one game of Halo and stop. The music and video stream calls them back to action, and they push the buttons and go—again, and again, and again. If you think about it, these are the games that never end. They stimulate pleasure centers of the brain for a brief period of time (the duration of a game) and then remind the child to push a button so that they can get "turned on" again. Over an incredibly brief period of time, children go from having never played to craving the action of these games. And if you've ever tried to cut off your child's supply to their video game drug (or Internet drug, or smartphone drug), you've experienced a reaction every bit as intense as that of a kid who's watching his parents flush their stash of pot, cocaine, or whatever down the toilet. So let's talk about changing this type of pattern and beginning to teach your child the values that really matter. Here's another story from our family that might help.

One day, I came home and found one of our sons fooling around with his mom's phone. Now maybe you have the latest hi-tech version of phones with Internet connections, but we don't. Our phones are the pathetic flip-phones that just do the phone thing. Anyway, our son picked up my wife's phone, which is probably the last of the flip phones ever created, but it does have a little game section, and one of the games is Ms. Pac-Man.

Ms. Pac-Man is not a big, high-action game. Just a little smiley face character, picking up little dots on a screen while trying to avoid ghosties. Well, my son had the intense look of a surgeon in a life-saving mission on his face as he worked the little buttons. I watched for a moment or two as he played, lost, played, lost, played, succeeded a little, and then lost again. I asked him to stop for a minute. Naturally, he ignored me, because boys are usually more anchored on sights than sounds. So I moved in and told him that he needed to pause the game. I said, "Can I have the game for a minute? I want to show you something."

Well, my son looked at me with one of those "uh-oh" faces, and I continued. I said to Diego, "Hey D, I want you to do something for me. I want you to play Ms. Pac-Man just one time then stop, and then tell me how you feel." So he did. When he was done, I asked him to look at me, and I asked him "Diego, how do you feel? Are you feeling happy? All full of joy and ready to play with me?" He shook his head and said, "No, Dad, I want to play again." No surprise, right? So I said, "OK, D, play it again, and see how you feel then." He did, and after he finished, I asked him if he felt "all full." Of course he said, "No, Dad, I want to play again." I told him, "All right, let's try it one more time and see if it fills you up." So he plays again, with the same result.

At that point, I sat face to face with Diego and shared one simple truth. I told him that the problem I have with video games is that they steal our time and never really satisfy us. No matter how many times you play, and no matter how many challenges you beat, you never really win, you never get to the end of the game, and you never get that "mmmmm" satisfied feeling. And after hours and hours, you haven't spent any real time with your family or friends and you haven't done anything that gives you a good feeling inside. So we put down the game, talked about the activities that gave us a good feeling, and headed downstairs to play some floor hockey together, which was a lot of fun and gave us the feeling we wanted (even though he beat me).

THE POWER OF POSITIVE PRACTICE

So let's take some time to talk about how you could begin to teach the traits that you really want your children to learn. Let's start by thinking about what you've learned about how to teach any new skill. First, you'll need to decide which of these traits (or others that you might think about) you'd like to teach. Then, you'll need to decide on a place and time that you'll introduce the idea to your child (remember the 10-second rule). And even though we're talking about "virtues" or "admirable traits," remember, most little kids and teens aren't instinctively generous, compassionate, and so on.

To help your child experience the joy that comes with learning these traits, you'll have to set the stage and use the kinds of motivational strategies that we've covered in this book. So decide on the trait that you want your children to learn, think about the kinds of positive practice and positive punishment techniques you'll use to teach and motivate your child, and look for the time to get started. Here are some examples of how some parents have started to teach values to their kids.

One parent decided that to teach *generosity* to a battling 6-year-old and his brother. There was no big lecture. The parent had decided that it was time for a change and told the boys it was time to start working on being generous and sharing. One day, the two little guys came into their house after school. They were both hungry and went to the cupboard for some Cheetos. Instead of finding two snack-size bags of this tasty treat, they found one. The first boy yelled, "Hey that's mine." The second said, "Hey, you had the last bag, this is mine." So the grappling started, and the parent said, "Wait a minute, both of you have a seat."

Now the parent could have said, "Because of how you acted, no one gets the Cheetos." The parent could have said, "No TV." Instead of a takeaway, an opportunity to feel what generosity was like was about to occur. It went like this. The parent said, "You boys have been yelling at each other over a bag of Cheetos. I want you to remember how that feels." After a brief pause, the parent took the bag of Cheetos and poured about half of the bag in front of each child. The boys were told to take turns asking their brother if he wanted a Cheeto. The brother was to say, "Yes, please." Then the child was to give his brother a Cheeto, and the brother was to say "Thank you." The parent watched as the boys started doing this, pretty awkwardly at first.

By the time the boys got halfway through their piles, they were laughing and giggling. When all of the Cheetos were gone, the parent just asked, "How did it feel to be generous and share?" By then, the mood was totally different, and the boys knew that it was because their parent had helped them reach in and pull out something better that was inside them. Instead of being selfish and greedy, they had experienced the joy of generosity. They liked it better. Pretty cool!

Now this is a pretty neat example of positive practice. For most of us, when our kids do something that we don't like, our first reaction is to yell, correct them, and take something away, like a toy, a TV show, a chance to play video games or go outside, or whatever the child likes. Psychologists call that *negative punishment* because we're trying to discourage our children from doing something we don't like by taking something away. In positive practice, a parent finds a way to teach a skill by having them practice handling the situation the "right way."

The use of positive practice is found everywhere. I think I learned a lot about this from my baseball-playing days. The coaches who taught me the most were the ones who knew that it wasn't yelling, threatening, or benching me that paid off. It was practicing the "right way." So one day, I was playing third base and missed four ground balls in a row. I was embarrassed and mad. My coach called my name; he wasn't yelling. I looked up, and he said, "Catch" and tossed a marble down the third base line. I caught it; he smiled and tossed me another. I caught that one too. He did it one more time, with the same result and then said, "Just wanted to make sure you remembered to get down on the ball. If you can catch a marble, you can catch anything." And I did.

Now we all know that one experience isn't necessarily transformational, but it is the beginning of the way toward developing a new skill or trait. Just like we make sure our children are learning to be responsible by getting their homework done, we can use self-ish moments, embarrassing moments, and angry moments to teach generosity, courage, and inner peace by practicing doing things the "right way." Let's look at one more example. This one is on *kindness and resilience.*

Most of us don't have to travel far to come face to face with a natural disaster. A few years ago, my hometown got hit really hard. On the first day of school in 2011, a heavy rain started to fall in the Binghamton, New York, area. By midday, rivers were rising, and the call was made to evacuate the schools. By the time busses were transporting kids home, some of the roadways were already flooded. Eventually, all of the kids made it home. Unfortunately, for thousands, home would soon be a distant memory.

Within a few hours, it was clear that this was going to be a big deal. In a day, we became a disaster area, and the sound of helicopters surveying the scene was commonplace. I personally had never seen anything like it in the town I call home. Neither had most of the other people in our region. Moments like these bring out the best and worst in us. Some of the parents of the kids in my clinic decided it would be a good time to teach kindness.

Instead of being content that their children were safe and their homes were undamaged, a number of the kids in my clinic were taught the good feeling that comes with kindness. With the guidance of their parents, they began to bring some of their toys for kids stuck in gymnasiums and other shelters. Others went to their churches and got involved in preparing meals for families who had been displaced. Teenagers went with their dads and moms to help with the endless process of tearing out waterlogged plaster, power washing and sanitizing basements and structures, and bringing a little hope and encouragement to people who had lost nearly all of their stuff. The parents could have just let these kids sit, watch TV, play their games, and go on with their lives. They didn't. And their kids got to experience the joy that comes from simply being kind. That's a lesson they will never learn surfing the Internet, blowing away a day on video games, or keeping up with Twitter, e-mails, and Facebook postings on their smartphones.

At the same time that these children were learning how good it feels to be kind, they were also learning about resilience. You see, the people who were receiving these acts of kindness weren't just sitting around moping. Yes, their homes were flooded from the basement to the ceiling of the first floor, porches were torn off, and cars were floating away. My neighbors were surely stunned, shocked, and saddened at first. But when the kids got to these areas, they didn't find people sitting and waiting to be rescued. They saw grown-ups and kids pulling the rotting debris out of their homes, piece by drenched piece. And even though the piles mounted high on the sidewalks and a yellowish, dusty haze clouded the streets, one simple fact couldn't be hidden: In the face of a shockingly destructive flood, one that cost people pretty much all that they owned, a community realized that what mattered wasn't stuff, but people. Their response to the disaster caused a straightforward "reset" of the value button for many of the kids and grown-ups who went in to help.

DON'T WAIT FOR DISASTER TO STRIKE

It goes without saying that you don't have to wait for a disaster to strike before you begin to teach traits such as resilience. So take a few moments to consider which traits you want to teach. Then begin to look for a chance to teach. Those moments will surely come. Just be ready to do something other than yell, preach, or take away. It doesn't matter what you begin with. What does matter is that during those once-a-week strategy meetings we discussed, you begin to think about those values that are important for your child to learn, and decide on your lesson plan.

At my clinic, I've heard of parents teaching their children to share their allowance. Instead of putting away some percentage of their allowance for their college education, I know parents who are teaching their children to set aside a 10th of their allowance to give to organizations that are dedicated to bringing drinking water to people in Africa, Asia, and South America. Some of the teenagers I know are being taught to use some of the money from their part-time jobs to fund the $38 per month that it takes to sponsor a child through organizations such as Compassion (www.compassion.com) so that a child in a poverty-stricken region of the world would have food, water, medical care, and education. When I've talked with my patients about what they experienced when their parents started teaching them these traits, it became clear that something transformational was happening. As you teach your children about big-picture values, I have no doubt that your kids will feel those life-changing moments too.

HOMEWORK

As you think about the next steps for your child, maybe it's time to consider focusing on what really matters. At our clinic, it's been pretty easy to encourage parents to take this step. What's amazing is how quickly children respond and how reinforcing it is for them. Unlike other kinds of desired or target behaviors, the experiences that children have when they are generous, kind, patient, resilient, or compassionate seem to be sufficiently reinforcing that you don't have to punish them (although you will need to introduce your children to the idea and guide them through positive practice). So pick a trait that you'd like to nurture, and enjoy this next step in the development of your child with ADHD.

LESSON 11

PARENTS ARE PEOPLE TOO!

In this lesson, I want to shift focus. Now that you understand that attention-deficit/hyperactivity disorder (ADHD) is a health problem (just like diabetes, anemia, and other medical conditions that can affect how a person acts), I hope you can use this knowledge and channel your energies into the gradual process of helping your child improve his or her behavior a little bit each day. I reviewed the importance of the careful use of medication and of maintaining a balanced diet that includes eating a sufficient amount of protein in the morning and at lunchtime. I talked about establishing family rules to teach kids that in life, you get what you work for. I examined strategies designed to promote your child's sensitivity by encouraging them to make amends when they make mistakes and to solve problems by learning about the needs and fears of others. Beyond these techniques and strategies, I encouraged you to consider thinking about teaching your children the values and virtues that really matter, and I stressed the importance of demonstrating to your child each and every day that she or he is loved and is special to you.

So, what about you? Chances are that since your child was born, you have spent many (if not all) of your waking hours trying to keep her or him out of harm's way. Trying to figure out strategies to help your child get organized, stay on top of responsibilities, remember what he or she has been told, and so on, and so on. In essence, you have played the role of your child's brain for as long as he or she has been alive. That is a draining job. When was the last time you sat down and planned some quality time for yourself to unwind? Let's think about that for a bit.

A long time ago, in a lifetime far, far away, you were just yourself. You were a person trying to figure out a way to survive, have some fun, and feel halfway decent about who you are. OK, so you're a bit older now. However, that doesn't change the fact that you still need to have a bit of fun and feel halfway decent about yourself. In this lesson, I share a couple of parent "antidepressant" activities for you to consider. I hope you take the lessons to heart. If you are physically and mentally drained, it is unlikely you'll have the strength to teach your child any of the lessons in this book.

SELF-CARE ACTIVITIES FOR ADULTS

1. Each Day, Do at Least Three Things Just Because You Like to Do Them

Let's start with this. I have to say that in my decades as a psychologist, I've heard many people tell me that they spend their days doing all sorts of things for other people and feel exhausted and massively depressed. So the first idea that I want you to consider is how every day you can do a couple of activities that you enjoy.

Typically, when people hear this, they think that I am out of touch with reality. No, I really don't think that a single mother of six kids is going to easily find a way (or the desire) to hit that abs class at the Y three nights a week. I mean, that's great if you can get coverage for the kids. What I'm talking about are the simple pleasures in life.

I'm talking about getting some help from your kids so you can watch your favorite TV show. I'm talking about munching on a warm bagel in the morning with peanut butter and honey on it. I'm talking about putting your favorite music on and listening to it while you work. I'm talking about reading a recreational or inspirational book during a break at work. I'm talking about going to one of those megabookstores (with or without the kids), settling into a chair, sipping on a mochaccino, and reading while the kids explore the world of books. I'm talking about visiting a friend in person, or through Facebook, e-mail, or by phone (how old school is that?). I'm talking about surfing the Internet. I'm talking about munching on some fries on the way home from work. I'm talking about a Snickers bar that you look forward to in the midafternoon. I'm talking about walking your dog, strolling through a park, hiking in the woods, biking to the store instead of driving. I can go on and on (my patients tell me that I certainly can), but I think you know what I mean. Be deliberate. Make a point of picking out three things you will do today just because you like them. Do this every day. Believe me, it helps.

2. Protein Is Important for Parents Too! Grab at Least 20 Grams for Breakfast and for Lunch

Let's be honest. You'll never make it on coffee, cigarettes, and donuts. There is no way that skipping protein at breakfast will gear you up for success. You know the routine. You're too busy with the kids to eat in the morning. So you gulp some coffee on the road. By 9:00 a.m., you hit the wall. You have another cup of coffee (or other caffeine drink), plus some carbs (donut, muffin). Perhaps you add some nicotine to the mix. Maybe you kid yourself and think that a glass of juice for breakfast will do the trick. That's a step in the right direction, but it's really just more sugar with none of the protein needed to fuel your decision-making brain. So far, your body has not consumed anywhere near the 20 to 30 grams of protein that you need in the morning. Chances are high that this afternoon, you'll feel mentally drained and physically fatigued. Not a great state to be in when you and the kids meet up again at home.

Maybe you couldn't care less about weight, so you pack it in at lunch. Megasized meal at Burger World. The foot-long sub, packed with cheese and meat. The leisurely lunch at the nearby pasta place, with huge servings of spaghetti and meatballs. If you've skipped or skimped at breakfast, these types of meals are likely to leave you mentally exhausted, and they certainly don't set the stage for effective functioning at work or at home.

The bottom line is that all the information about the importance of protein at breakfast and at lunch isn't just for the kids. Grab a soy-based protein shake if your appetite is low in the morning. Hate the taste of soy? Go for a whey-based shake. Still too much mass? Remember those Gatorade G-3 drinks or Ensure's light berry-flavored protein drinks with a Special K protein bar or a Cliff Bar.

Not a shake person? That's OK. Boil a bunch of eggs at night and store them in the fridge. You can munch on a couple in the morning. Hey, you don't even need to eat the yolk (the protein's in the whites). In a time crunch? Roll up a little boiled ham, chicken breast, or turkey breast with a slice of cheese and walk out the door munching. Not only will these strategies help you feel awake in the morning at work, they'll prevent the fatigue that hits many of us after lunch. Besides, feeling well is part of the plan for you!

3. Everybody Needs a Dream (Even Parents)

I believe it was those famous philosophers the Rolling Stones who once sang, "lose your dreams and you will lose your mind." I think there's something to that one. Part of what keeps us feeling alive is staying true to your version of the big picture. Here's antidepressant idea Number 3: Make a wish list. Here are a dozen prompts to get you started. Complete the sentences with whatever comes to mind:

If I weren't so old, I'd like to _____

Before I'm "over the hill," I want to _____

If I wasn't so afraid, I'd _____

Even though it's silly, I like _____

If I had an extra $100, I'd _____

I sure would like it if my dad and I could _____

I sure would like it if my mom and I could _____

I sure would like it if my spouse or friend and I could _____

I always wanted to teach my kid to _____

I always wanted to learn to _____

When I look around my house or apartment, I wish I had the energy to _____

I think that it's important for me to always remember that

_____

_____

These aren't the only prompts you can use, but try these and see what happens. Beginning something new provides a source of energy that can make life much less burdensome.

4. Save Some Time for Those You Love

If you are married, are involved in a loving relationship, are close to members of your extended family, are a member of a church family, or have long-term friendships, make sure you cherish these connections. These are important sources of energy that will keep you afloat in tough times. Here are a few suggestions on how to keep these connections alive.

- Each day, ask yourself: "What did I do to show my spouse, love, friend, or other loved one that they are important to me?" Just as we need three meals of food every day, your spouse or loved one could use three "love meals" too. Think about what spells love to your spouse or loved one (ask if you need to, it's OK). A lot of us walk around feeling unappreciated for our efforts. It's often not appreciated because it didn't translate to love to others. Working in a factory all day long might be your way of saying "I love you" to your family, but your wife might spell love as, "he tucks the kids in at night so I can finish the laundry." Think about it. Find a way to do three acts that actually mean love to someone you love. You'll be amazed with the results.

- Each week, spend part of at least one day alone with your "love" doing something that the two of you enjoy. It doesn't matter if it boils down to munching on a bowl of popcorn while watching reruns of *The Andy Griffith Show* or *Friends* (one of my and my wife's favorite evening activities). It doesn't matter if you just sit quietly together and ask each other, "What else can I do to show you I love you?" What counts is that the two of you are together, and it's your time to enjoy as you please.

- Each season, try to go on an overnight trip away from the kids. Because we all need this kind of rejuvenation, relatives and friends often exchange babysitting for each other. Even one night away somewhere close to home is rejuvenating, and it's easier to get coverage for the kids if it's close by and you're only going away for one night.

- Kindness, compassion, and generosity create energy too. Most of us realize that, but when we get fatigued, those joyous memories can fade. As we talked about in the previous lesson, getting your family engaged in random acts of kindness, compassion, and generosity is energizing. In our family, even simple events such as Halloween have been transformed. Several days before Halloween, we sneak out and visit a couple of houses. We'll put a little ghost sign on their door that says "You've Been Booed" (you can get these online at www.BeenBooed.com). The next day, we'll make some goodies and treats for their family and return the night before Halloween and drop them off (ring the bell) and take off. Our kids love doing this one. On Halloween, our family will spend part of the afternoon baking muffins, cookies, and other treats for our neighbors. When my little guys go trick-or-treating, they're bringing the goodies, as well as getting some. At Christmastime, my sons accompany me and my wife when we visit nursing homes to sing carols and spread some love. You can imagine the smiles on the faces of people when my 8-year-old sons say "Merry Christmas" and hands them a candy cane. Neater still are the smiles and memories that are being created inside us and our boys. So let yourself and your kids begin to think about joining in and creating random acts of kindness.

5. Rediscover Your Moral Compass

When I spoke with you about the sources of self-confidence in a child, I mentioned the connection between self-esteem and a person's moral code. Most of us have made choices because of pleasure, despair, anxiety, and rage that run absolutely counter to our moral code. And even though it can be too late to change those choices, it is never too late to rediscover your moral compass and begin setting a new life course that matches your beliefs. It is rare to find a person who has no regrets, and yet the burden that can come from living under the weight of constant reminders of how you blew it and made mistakes can get in the way of you raising successful, confident kids who can take responsibilities for their mistakes, regroup, apologize, make amends, and move forward. So if you're feeling weighed down by a sense of guilt over poor life choices, do what you've begun to teach your children: Apologize, find a way to make amends, and begin to live a life that matches your moral code.

6. Don't Isolate Yourself and Try to Raise Kids With ADHD Without Help

There are some tasks in life that we can't do alone. Successfully raising kids with ADHD is one of them. To help your child succeed at home, at school, on the playground, and eventually in the workplace and in adult relationships, you need assistance. Establishing relationships with health care professionals who are knowledgeable about the various types of treatments needed by children with ADHD is an important first step. If the only type of treatment your child is receiving is medication, then you need to identify other resources in your community. As I stress throughout this book, there are many, many lessons medications cannot teach.

A good place to start is by asking your child's pediatrician for recommendations for a psychologist or other mental health professional who specializes in the treatment of ADHD. Another useful strategy is to contact the national organization for individuals with ADHD (Children and Adults With Attention-Deficit/Hyperactivity Disorder, or CHADD; see www.chadd.org). CHADD provides educational materials and can assist you in learning about local chapters that conduct educational and support meetings. Both the national and local CHADD organizations can help you learn about support groups in your community. Members of these groups are also likely to be able to provide the names of individuals who specialize in the treatment of ADHD. Such individuals will be able to assist you in developing a treatment plan for your child that is much more comprehensive than medication alone.

If you are unable to locate a specialist in your region through support groups, a university medical center may be helpful. Most university-based medical centers have child and adolescent psychiatrists and psychologists who either treat kids with ADHD or can assist you in identifying such specialists near you. Another resource that can help you locate a specialist is a graduate program in clinical psychology or social work at a college or university near your community.

Finally, the Internet makes networking with other parents who have children with ADHD is easier than ever. I've also found that magazines such as *ADDitude* (www.additude.com) provide a lot of information and ways to connect with others. Having friends who know what it's like, firsthand, can be a real blessing too.

HOMEWORK

Homework? What homework? This lesson was about some R & R for you. Take a little time for yourself. Remember that simple pleasures can be the best!

IT DON'T COME EASY: TROUBLESHOOTING TIPS

Whenever I finish reading a parenting book, I typically have a sense that something is missing. No matter how sensible the advice, no matter how practical the ideas, I recognize that the learning process is not easy. You know that too. I usually find myself wondering, "Is it really that easy?" Well, at this point, you have almost finished reading my parenting book. However, it is unlikely that your child is "all better." I hope that some of the lessons shared in this book are taking hold. Maybe your child isn't as prone to anger. Maybe he is doing better in school. Maybe it doesn't take a dozen reminders for her to do what she is supposed to do. However, the odds are that your child still whines, gripes, loses his cool, and at times tries to avoid tasks that require sustained mental effort. So it makes little sense to pretend that when parents complete my 10-session program all is well.

Having taught hundreds of parent groups this program, I recognize that most parents have difficulties putting lessons into action. Chances are, so will you. In this lesson, I share some of the common problems experienced by parents in my program and offer ideas for overcoming them. Let's start by reviewing where you are in the change process.

When you began reading this book, you completed a list of improvements that you wanted to see in your child. Since that time, I hope you've learned about the causes of attention-deficit/hyperactivity disorder (ADHD), the importance of nutrition, the need for a supportive educational plan, the benefits of medication and attention-training programs, as well as other strategies to improve the lives of children and teens with ADHD. Mort important, I ask that you think about the quality of your family life and how children learn new skills.

In this book, I emphasize that learning requires several steps. First, you must plan what you want to teach and give the child advance notice. Second, you should not try to teach a new lesson in the middle of a conflict situation. Third, the child needs to be told (simply and directly) what you want him or her to do or not do. Fourth, the child needs to realize that if he or she does not do what is required by you, there will be specific consequences (most commonly, that life is on hold until the child does what was requested and something in addition to practice and make up for the behavior). Fifth, if the child displayed anger toward you, was disrespectful, or whined and gave you a hard time, he or she needs to apologize, do some kind of make up, and then follow your directions.

When we considered the lessons you wanted to teach your child, I asked you to analyze your lesson plan and think about the sequence of events that took place. What did you say to your child? What did the child do? What were the consequences of his or her actions? So often children persist in their old ways by arguing, whining, avoiding, and refusing to cooperate. If the result of the defiance or avoidance leads you to back off and the child does not have to comply, no improvement will occur. As one little boy told me, "Why should I do what my parents want me to do? If I do, they only ask me to do more. If I don't, they just go away and ask my brother to do it, or do it themselves." Time and again, I have seen that no change occurs in the child if the parents were not clear about what they wanted or if there were no consequences for the child's actions (other than some parent lecture).

In this book, I ask you to reflect on your family life and what you really want to teach your children. I stress the importance of setting aside some time each day to give your child the gift of your attention. I ask you to consider establishing a "nonaggression pact" in your family so your home can become a place where aggression, teasing, and sarcasm are not OK. I also emphasize the importance of weekly parent planning time, a scheduled time when you think about what you are trying to teach and what changes need to be made in your lesson plan. I ask you to consider teaching your child how to solve problems by learning to discover the concerns and needs of others. Finally, I discuss the obvious fact that if you are going to be an effective parent, you need love, companionship, fun, and a healthy diet. So my question now is: How are you doing? Is your family moving in the right direction? I hope so. However, chances are there is still room for improvement. Take a few minutes and complete the Parenting Program Checklist. It should give you a better idea what needs to be done now.

Now that you've finished the questionnaire, let's look at your answers. If you are following treatment plan recommendations for "The Basics" and "Parent Self-Care" but are having specific "Skill Development Problems," take a few minutes to consider your lesson plan. For those skills that are not progressing, have you told your child what is required? Are you using motivational strategies such as Time Stands Still, combined with apologies and amends? If not, meet with your child, review your lesson plan, and start again.

If you are not following treatment plan recommendations for "The Basics" and "Parent Self-Care" sections, welcome to the club. These are the two areas where parenting efforts often bog down. However, they cannot be ignored if you are to succeed in your efforts

Parenting Program Checklist

(Place a check under Yes or No)

Treatment Plan: The Basics	YES	NO
My child has been evaluated by a physician for other medical problems that can cause "ADHD" symptoms.	——	——
My child has been evaluated for visual problems (acuity, tracking, and convergence) by an optometrist or ophthalmologist and for auditory problems by an audiologist.	——	——
My child is being treated for ADHD with medication, EEG biofeedback, and/or computerized attention training.	——	——
My child eats at least 20 grams of protein:		
At breakfast	——	——
At lunch	——	——
My child sleeps at least 8 hours per night.	——	——
My child has been referred for evaluation by the Committee on Special Education and an IEP or 504 Plan has been established (or is in the process of being developed).	——	——
My family has agreed to the Parent–Child Non-aggression Pact.	——	——
I plan weekly meetings to review goals for my children and revise my parenting plan, as needed.	——	——

Treatment Plan: Skill Development	YES	NO
My child follows family rules:		
Before school	——	——
After school	——	——
After dinner	——	——
When my child doesn't follow family rules or displays inappropriately intense anger, sadness, or anxiety I		
use Time Stands Still.	——	——
Insist on an apology.	——	——

Parenting Program Checklist *(Continued)*

Require them to "practice" the right way. _____ _____

Require them to do something extra to make up for their actions. _____ _____

Treatment Plan: Skill Development
                                                    YES   **NO**

My child solves problems by asking about my concerns and needs and "brainstorms" with me to find a solution. _____ _____

My child is involved in activities that matter to his or her peers. _____ _____

My child engages in conversations about topics of interest to others. _____ _____

My child records daily activities and responsibilities on a board, book, cell phone, or other visual prompt. _____ _____

I spend at least 15 minutes each day enjoying a recreational activity with my child. _____ _____

I am encouraging my child to develop at least one social value or "virtue" (e.g., generosity, compassion, kindness). _____ _____

Treatment Plan: Parent "Self-Care"

I do three things that I enjoy every day. _____ _____

I eat at least 20 grams of protein:
  At breakfast _____ _____
  At lunch _____ _____

I am currently working on achieving one of my "dreams." _____ _____

I show my partner that she or he is loved by me in ways that "count" to my partner. _____ _____

I sleep at least 7 hours per day. _____ _____

© Vincent J. Monastra

to help your child. The following are some common problems experienced by the parents who have participated in my parenting classes, along with some suggestions on what to do about them.

Problem 1: Your child continues to demonstrate poor response to first-line treatments for ADHD (i.e., stimulant medications) and does not seem to be learning much from your efforts to use the lessons in this book.

Suggestion: Make sure that your child has been tested for other conditions listed on the questionnaire and that you have addressed dietary and sleep problems. If you have ignored this important step, please reconsider. Before you start combining medications, shifting to "non-ADHD" medications, or concluding that your child is emotionally disturbed, have your child tested (and treated) for other medical conditions and address any dietary or sleep problems.

Problem 2: Your child is not responding to stimulant medications, but there are no other medical, nutritional, or sleep issues. The physician has increased the dose, but that appears to be making the situation worse.

Suggestion: Consider a quantitative electroencephalographic (QEEG) evaluation for your child. Published studies conducted by my clinic as well as research centers in the United States, Canada, Europe, and Australia have noted that underactivity in the frontal and central midline regions of the brain is a common characteristic of patients with ADHD who respond to methylphenidate-based medications. However, this research has indicated that approximately 10% to 20% of patients with ADHD do not demonstrate such underactivity and do not respond well to methylphenidate-based medications. An alternative to a trial-and-error strategy would be to conduct a QEEG evaluation. If underactivity is not apparent on a QEEG, a mixed amphetamine salt (e.g., Adderall), a nonstimulant ADHD medication (Strattera), or an antihypertensive medication (e.g., Catapres, Tenex, Intuniv) alone or in combination with a low dose of a mixed amphetamine salt may prove helpful. Discuss these options with your child's prescribing physician.

Problem 3: Your child appears to be improving with medication but is still not completing schoolwork or homework and is disruptive in class. The school district thinks that your child is lazy and is resistant to conducting an evaluation.

Suggestion: Write a letter to the chairperson of the Committee on Special Education or to whoever is responsible for conducting evaluations and coordinating the development of Individualized Education Plans (IEPs) and 504 Plans in your child's school district. Inform them that your child has been diagnosed with ADHD (provide written documentation by the health care provider who made the diagnosis). Request that an evaluation for learning disabilities and functional impairments associated with ADHD be conducted (as mandated by the educational laws in every state). The district must respond to such a written request. After the evaluation is completed, an IEP or 504 Plan will be developed to help with any learning disabilities or functional problems. However, these plans do not address motivational issues, or the deterioration of medication effects in the late afternoon and early evening, when many children are beginning to do their homework. Assistance may be provided at school in the form of resource room teachers who can make sure that assignments are recorded and materials organized and brought home, but such help doesn't really address the child's lack of motivation and limited ability to concentrate as medications wear off.

To address such problems, I have several suggestions. First, I strongly recommend that parents be informed on the day that any assignment is not completed and turned in. Most schools have e-mail contact information for parents, which is the easiest way. If necessary, a phone call could be made. Without learning about missing homework on the day due, parents cannot begin to address the motivational or medical causes of the missing assignments.

Second, if a child fails to turn in an assignment, then he or she needs to complete the missing assignment plus a similar one designed by the parents or teacher in the same subject area. If the child does not have the worksheet or "forgot" the nature of the assignment, parents should assign two school tasks of their choice (e.g., two sheets of math problems for a missing math paper, reading about a historical event or person, or a scientific fact or discovery, and then writing an essay on the topic). If the teachers are unable to give such a daily accounting of missing work, then a weekly progress report is needed. That report will need to specify the exact nature of the assignment so that it can be completed over the weekend. Any assignments listed as incomplete on the weekly progress report must be done before the child can engage in enjoyable recreational activities on the weekend (Time Stands Still). They'll also need to be assigned some extra schoolwork to "inspire" them to get the work done on time (positive practice). And if they get mad, whine, or the like, they'll need to make up with you by doing something nice for you (positive punishment).

Third, if a pattern of incomplete assignments is noted, you should consult with your child's physician or psychologist to discuss the need for a booster dose of medication in the afternoon. I have found that a number of children simply do not have the attention and concentration abilities to do homework after dinner, and the fights can be horrible. To address the medical issue, a booster dose of an immediate-release type of stimulant (e.g., Ritalin, Focalin, Adderall) could be administered after lunch or right after school (3 p.m.). Such a booster may provide sufficient improvement of attention to get the work done.

Finally, because an ounce of prevention is often worth a pound of cure, I have found it very helpful to make arrangements for homework to be done before the child gets home after school. This can be done in several ways. For middle and high school students, I find that having a study hall plus a resource room is often sufficient to complete homework. It makes much more sense for high school students with ADHD to have such periods and actually pass their subjects than to eliminate study halls so that they can magically complete their high school requirements in 3 years and spend their senior year earning college credits. When schedule restrictions make that difficult, some school districts have Homework Clubs or an extra period for the child to work with a teacher and get work done. Boys & Girls Clubs of America, YMCAs, churches, and other social agencies also offer Homework Clubs in some communities.

Don't have access to such programs? Think about making arrangements for a high school student, college student, or one of the thousands of unemployed teachers with master's degrees to meet with your child at a library, Starbucks, Barnes & Noble, or other public place. For far less than the cost of a single counseling session with a psychologist or other health care provider to talk about the problem of missing homework and the battles at home, you could hire a tutor to work with your child 4 days a week and take care of the problem. Think about it.

Problem 4: Everything seems to be going along fine until the evening. There appear to be no adverse effects because of your child's use of a sustained-release stimulant medication during the daytime. However, at night your child is arguing, throwing tantrums, refusing to follow your rules, and won't go to sleep.

Suggestion: There are medical, nutritional, and psychological strategies to consider. Medical interventions that seem to help with this type of problem include use of antihypertensive medications (e.g., Catapres, Tenex) in the evening to reduce aggression and promote sleep onset. Monitoring dietary habits may reveal that your child is not eating sufficient protein at breakfast or lunch (reducing the ability to manufacture brain "sedating" neurotransmitters at night) or continues to drink caffeinated beverages at night. Increasing protein intake at breakfast and lunch and eliminating consumption of caffeinated drinks after dinner may be helpful. Parenting strategies (e.g., needing to apologize and do some type of corrective action before being allowed to play that night or the next afternoon) may also help.

Problem 5: You are arguing with your child all the time (or at least it feels that way) and are too overwhelmed to schedule a parent meeting to think about what you should do.

Suggestion: Let's start with some basic care for you. If you are "relapsing" and arguing like crazy, nothing positive is going to happen until you get that squared away. So trust that good ideas for helping your child will come to mind after you get some rest, start eating 20 grams of protein at breakfast and lunch, and begin doing things that you enjoy each day. One of my favorite acronyms from Alcoholics Anonymous is HALT (Hungry, Angry, Lonely, Tired). Essentially, the idea is that a person will relapse into old, destructive habits when he or she is hungry, angry, lonely, or tired. You're only human. If you are feeling as though things are out of control, begin with yourself and start to address your hunger, anger, loneliness, and fatigue. Then return to this book, review those lessons that cover the skill development areas you want to work on, and get started. If this doesn't work and you continue to feel overwhelmed, schedule an appointment for yourself with your doctor. There may be undiagnosed medical problems that are getting in the way. Or, as you may have suspected, you too may have ADHD and need effective treatment.

FINAL THOUGHTS:
A PERSONAL PERSPECTIVE

It's been said that if you see a turtle sitting on a fence post, you can be sure that he didn't get there all by himself. The same is true for book authors. There is no way that we could learn the information that we share in books by ourselves. So I'd like to express my gratitude to those who helped me, and I thought you might like to know who they are.

First, I want to thank my wife, Donna. It has been said that with love, all things are possible. Simply put, without her love, encouragement, and support, the second edition of my parenting book would not have been written. She encouraged me to take on this project and tolerated the endless hours apart while I worked on the manuscript. She also served as the first editor of this book, helping me to incorporate new developments in our clinical program into the lessons taught in this book. It was largely because of her editing efforts that the complexities of attention-deficit/hyperactivity disorder were translated into words that could be easily understood and put into practice. I also want to thank Susan Herman for her insightful guidance throughout the completion of this book, as well as the production team at the American Psychological Association for bringing this book to press.

I also want to express my thanks to my parents. Although both of my parents were somewhat apologetic that they had never gone to college, they possessed wisdom and the kind of common sense that has served me well. My mom was the person who taught me the value of Work for Play, and it was my dad's patience in the midst of turmoil that served as my model for the problem-solving strategies I use in my clinical work. I'll never forget sitting at the kitchen table going over options to solve a problem as he jotted down ideas on a dinner napkin.

Next, I'd like to express my appreciation to my professors, supervisors, and mentors, beginning with Dr. Paul Toomin, who taught me that scientific research requires more than a series of "pilot" studies. I'd also like to thank Dr. Doug Lowe, who introduced me to the world of psychophysiology, and brain–behavior relationships, and Dr. Joel Lubar, who showed me how the brains of patients with ADHD could begin to heal through electroencephalographic biofeedback. I'd also like to express my appreciation to the training staff at the Philadelphia Child Guidance Clinic for helping me develop my skills in parent counseling and family therapy. I'll never forget my predawn drives to the Children's Hospital of Philadelphia, the countless late-night hours viewing videotapes of treatment sessions, and the opportunity to learn from Dr. Salvador Minuchin, Dr. Carl Whitaker, Dr. Ken Covelman, Barbara Forbes-Bryant, Jamshed Morenas, Jorge Colapinto, and the rest of the highly talented and greatly respected staff.

I'd also like to express my appreciation to my patients and their parents for having the courage to believe that change was possible, despite years of disappointment and frustration. I truly believe that my patients with ADHD are the nation's diamonds in the rough. They are extraordinary individuals who have the potential to make significant contributions to our society, if they can make it through the primary and secondary grades with their confidence and self-esteem intact. My job, and yours, is to make sure that they are not discarded.

Finally, I want to thank God for giving me the ability to learn certain truths and share them with others. It's ironic that when I think about those "discoveries" I've made in my clinical research, I realize that the most important ones were already written about several thousand years ago in a book called the Bible. Examples of Time Stands Still, positive practice, positive punishment, apologies, and amends abound in the Bible and can be found in other inspirational books as well. Sometimes we make it harder for ourselves by failing to take the time to consider what God's been trying to teach us forever. I'm grateful that through my conversations with the thousands of parents and children who came to visit me, these lessons hit home. I can only hope that the lessons I've learned will help you as your raise your child.

SUPPLEMENTAL RESOURCES

In this section, I provide a listing of video and audio programs, as well as books and scientific articles that can provide more detailed information about topics covered in each particular lesson. Most of the books are pretty easy reads, but if you are interested in learning more about the scientific research on a specific topic, you can find the papers that are listed (and many, many more) through PubMed (www.ncbi.nlm.nih.gov/pubmed). If you decide to search for information on PubMed, just enter key words such as *ADHD medication side effects*, *ADHD sleep disorders*, *ADHD diet*, or whatever topic you're interested in. PubMed will provide a list of scientific articles on the topic you've chosen, often with access to the complete articles.

The following supplemental readings have been separated by lesson number so you can easily find further readings on subjects covered in each lesson.

AUDIO AND VIDEO PROGRAMS BY DR. MONASTRA

Working With Children With ADHD (2005)

This DVD demonstrates the process of evaluating children with ADHD and includes parent–child counseling sessions. Available through the American Psychological Association (www.apa.org).

Parenting Children With ADHD: The Home Program (2010)

This 10-DVD set allows parents, health care providers, and parenting groups to watch the entire 10-class parenting program. Each DVD shows Dr. Monastra conducting and offering commentary as he teaches a different lesson live. The Home Program also includes the handouts used at our clinic to help parents complete homework assignments. Available through www.drvincemonastra.com.

Teaching Life Skills to Children With ADHD: The Home Program (2012)

This DVD set gives parents and their children the opportunity to learn life skills at home or with their counselor. Each DVD shows Dr. Monastra conducting and offering commentary as he teaches a different life skill live. The Home Program of the Life Skills Class also includes the handouts used at our clinic to help children complete homework assignments. Available through www. drvincemonastra.com.

"Get Focused"

This radio program features Dr. Monastra and his wife, Donna, offering practical solutions to problems facing adults and children in 21st century America from psychological, medical, and spiritual perspectives. Archives of these programs can be heard at any time by visiting www.timetofocus.org or at "Get Focused" on blogtalkradio.

SUPPLEMENTAL READINGS

The following books and scientific articles provide more detailed information about the scientific foundations of my parenting program. They are arranged by lesson to help you locate the information you are seeking more easily.

Introduction

Monastra, V. J. (2008). *Unlocking the potential of patients with ADHD: A model for clinical practice.* Washington, DC: American Psychological Association.

Monastra, V. J., Monastra, D., & George, S. (2002). The effects of stimulant therapy, EEG biofeedback, and parenting style on the primary symptoms of attention-deficit/hyperactivity disorder. *Applied Psychophysiology and Biofeedback, 27,* 231–249.

Lesson I

American Psychiatric Association. (2013). *The diagnostic and statistical manual of mental disorders* (5th ed.). Washington, DC: Author.

Monastra, V. J. (2008). *Unlocking the potential of patients with ADHD: A model for clinical practice.* Washington, DC: American Psychological Association.

National Institutes of Health. (1998, November). Diagnosis and treatment of attention deficit hyperactivity disorder. Consensus Development Conference Statement. Retrieved from http://consensus.nih.gov/1998/1998AttentionDeficitHyperactivityDisorder110html.htm

Lesson 2

Amen, D. G. (1998). *Change your brain, change your life.* New York, NY: Times Books.

Arns, M., Conners, K., & Kraemer, H. (2013). A decade of EEG theta/beta ratio research: A meta-analysis. *Journal of Attention Disorders, 17,* 374–383.

Barkley, R. A. (2005). *Attention-deficit/hyperactivity disorder: A handbook for diagnosis and treatment* (3rd ed.). New York, NY: Guilford Press.

Dougherty, D. D., Bonab, A. A., Spencer, T. J., Rauch, S. L., Madras, B. K., & Fishman, A. J. (1999). Dopamine transporter density in patients with attention deficit hyperactivity disorder. *Lancet, 354,* 1461–1462.

Giedd, J. N., Blumenthal, J., Molloy, E., & Castellanos, F. X. (2001). Brain imaging of attention deficit/hyperactivity disorder. *Annals of the New York Academy of Sciences, 931,* 33–49.

Monastra, V. J., Lubar, J. F., & Linden, M. (2001). The development of a quantitative electroencephalographic scanning process for attention-deficit/hyperactivity disorder: Reliability and validity studies. *Neuropsychology, 15,* 136–144.

Monastra, V. J., Lubar, J. F., Linden, M., VanDeusen, P., Green, G., Wing, W., . . . Fenger, T. N. (1999). Assessing attention-deficit/hyperactivity disorder via quantitative electroencephalography: An initial validation study. *Neuropsychology, 13,* 424–433.

Snyder, S. M., & Hall, J. R. (2006). A meta-analysis of quantitative electroencephalographic power associated with attention-deficit hyperactivity disorder. *Journal of Clinical Neurophysiology, 23,* 441–456.

Snyder, S. M., Quintana, H., Sexson, S. B., Knott, P., Haque, A. F. M., & Reynolds, D. A. (2008). Blinded, multi-center validation of EEG and rating scales in identifying ADHD within a clinical sample. *Psychiatry Research, 159,* 346–358.

Swanson, J. M., & Castellanos, F. X. (2002). Biological bases of ADHD: Neuroanatomy, genetics and pathophysiology. In P. S. Jensen & J. R. Cooper (Eds.), *Attention deficit hyperactivity disorder: State of the science: Best practices* (pp. 7-1–7-20). Kingston, NJ: Civic Research Institute.

Online Sources for Information on Quantitative Electroencephalographic Testing.

Tavernise, S. (2013, July 15). Brain test to diagnose A.D.H.D. is approved. Retrieved from www.nytimes.com/2013/07/16/health/brain-test-to-diagnose-adhd-is-approved.html

U.S. Food and Drug Administration. (2013, July 15). FDA permits marketing of first brain wave test to help assess children and teens for ADHD. Retrieved from www.fda.gov/newsevents/newsroom/pressannouncements/ucm360811.htm

www.accessdata.fda.gov/cdrh_docs/pdf

Lesson 3

American Academy of Pediatrics. (2013). *Evidence-based child and adolescent psychosocial interventions.* Retrieved from www.aap.org/mentalhealth

Arns, M., deRidder, S., Strehl, U., Breteler, M., & Coenen, A. (2009). Efficacy of neurofeedback treatment in ADHD: The effects on inattention, impulsivity, and hyperactivity: A meta-analysis. *Clinical EEG & Neuroscience, 40*, 180–189.

Chabot, R. J., Orgill, A. A., Crawford, G., Garris, M., & Serfontein, G. (1999). Behavioral and electrophysiologic predictors of treatment response to stimulants in children with attention disorders. *Journal of Child Neurology, 14*, 343–351.

Clarke, A. R., Barry, R. J., McCarthy, R., & Selikowitz, M. (2002). EEG differences between good and poor responders to methylphenidate and dexamphetamine in children with attention-deficit/hyperactivity disorder. *Clinical Neurophysiology, 113*, 194–205.

Loo, S. K., Hopfer, C., Teale, P. D., & Reite, M. (2004). EEG correlates of methylphenidate response in ADHD: Association with cognitive and behavioral measures. *Journal of Clinical Neurophysiology, 21*, 457–464.

McNab, F., Varrone, A., Fades, L., Jucaite, A., Bystritsky, P., Forssberg, H., & Klingberg, T. (2009). Changes in cortical dopamine D1 receptor binding associated with cognitive training. *Science, 323*, 800–802.

Melby-Lervaq, M., & Hulme, C. (2012). Is working memory training effective? A meta-analytic review. *Developmental Psychology, 49*, 270–291.

Monastra, V. J. (2005). Overcoming the barriers to effective treatment for attention-deficit/hyperactivity disorder: A neuro-educational approach. *International Journal of Psychophysiology, 58*, 71–80.

Monastra, V. J., & Lubar, J. F. (2013). *Neurofeedback in the treatment of attention-deficit/hyperactivity disorder* (4th ed.). In M. S. Schwartz & F. Andrasik (Eds.), *Biofeedback: A practitioner's guide.* New York, NY: Guilford Press.

Pelham, W. E. (2002). Psychosocial interventions for ADHD. In P. S. Jensen & J. R. Cooper (Eds.), *Attention deficit hyperactivity disorder: State of the science: Best practices* (pp. 12-2–12-36). Kingston, NJ: Civic Research Institute.

Rabiner, D. L., Murray, D. W., Skinner, A. T., & Malone, P. S. (2010) A randomized trial of two promising computer-based interventions for students with attention difficulties. *Journal of Abnormal Child Psychology, 38*, 131–142.

Wilens, T. E. (2004). *Straight talk about psychiatric medications for kids.* New York, NY: Guilford Press.

Lesson 4

Bruner, A. B., Joffe, A., Duggan, A. K., Casella, J. R., & Brandt, T. (1996). Randomized study of cognitive effects of iron supplementation in non-anemic, iron-deficit adolescent girls. *Lancet, 348,* 992–996.

Burgess, J. R., Stevens, L., Zhang, W., & Peck, L. (2000). Long-chain polyunsaturated fatty acids in children with attention-deficit hyperactivity disorder. *American Journal of Clinical Nutrition, 71,* 327–330.

Carlson, N. R. (2010). *Physiology of behavior* (10th ed.). Boston, MA: Allyn & Bacon.

Feingold, B. F. (1975). *Why your child is hyperactive.* New York, NY: Random House.

Fernstrom, J. D. (1983). Role of precursor availability in control of monamine biosynthesis in the brain. *Physiology Review, 63,* 485–546.

Fernstrom, J. D. (1994). Dietary amino acids and brain function. *Journal of the American Dietetic Association, 94,* 71–77.

Fernstrom, J. D. (1999). Effects of dietary polyunsaturated fatty acids on neuronal function. *Lipids, 34,* 161–169.

Fierke, C. (2000). Function and mechanism of zinc. *Journal of Nutrition, 130,* 1437S–1446S.

Fischer, K., Colombani, P. C., Langhans, W., & Wenk, C. (2001). Cognitive performance and its relationship with postprandial metabolic changes after ingestion of different macronutrients in the morning. *British Journal of Nutrition, 85,* 393–405.

Hambridge, M. (2000). Human zinc deficiency. *The Journal of Nutrition, 130*(Suppl. 5), 1344S–1349S.

Hartsough, C. S., & Lambert, N. M. (1985). Medical factors in hyperactive and normal children: Prenatal, developmental and health history findings. *American Journal of Orthopsychiatry, 55,* 190–210.

Kozielec, T., & Starobrat-Hermelin, B. (1994). Deficiency of certain trace elements in children with hyperactivity. *Polish Journal of Psychiatry, 28,* 345–353.

Rowe, K. S., & Rowe, K. J. (1994). Synthetic food coloring and behavior. A dose response effect in a double-blind, placebo-controlled, repeated-measures study. *The Journal of Pediatrics, 125,* 691–698.

Schmidt, M. H., Mocks, P., Lay, B., Eisert, H. G., Fojkar, R., Fritz-Sigmund, D., . . . Musaeus, B. (1997). Does oligoantigenic diet influence hyperactive/conduct-disordered children: A controlled trial. *European Child and Adolescent Psychiatry, 6,* 88–95.

Soniga-Barke, E. J., Brandeis, D., Cortese, S., Daley, D., Ferrin, M., Holtmann, M., . . . Sergeant, J.; European ADHD Guidelines Group. (2013). Nonpharmacological interventions for ADHD: Systematic review and meta-analyses of randomized controlled trials of dietary and psychological treatments. *American Journal of Psychiatry, 170,* 275–289.

Swanson, J. M., & Kinsbourne, M. (1980). Food dyes impair performance of hyperactive children on a laboratory learning test. *Science, 207,* 1485–1486.

Turer, C. B., Lin, H., & Flores, G. (2013). Prevalence of vitamin D deficiency among overweight and obese US children. *Pediatrics, 131,* 152–161.

Wurtman, R. J., & Wurtman, J. (Eds.). (1983). *Nutrition and the brain.* New York, NY: Raven Press.

Lesson 5

Cole, D., & Hallowell, E. M. (2000). *Learning outside the lines: Two Ivy League students with learning disabilities and ADHD give you the tools for academic success and educational revolution.* New York, NY: Simon & Schuster.

Mamary, A. (2007). *Creating the ideal school: Where teachers want to teach & students want to learn.* Lanham, MD: Rowman & Littlefield Education.

Teel, S. (2009). *Defending and parenting children who learn differently: Lessons from Edison's mother.* New York, NY: R & L.

Wending, B. J., & Mather, N. (2011). *Essentials of evidence-based academic interventions.* New York, NY: Wiley.

Lesson 6

Cooper, J. O., Heron, T. E., & Heward, W. L. (2007). *Applied behavior analysis.* Upper Saddle River, NJ: Pearson Education.

Weisz, J. R., & Kazdin, A. E. (2010). *Evidence-based psychotherapies for children and adolescents* (2nd ed.). New York, NY: Guilford Press.

Lesson 7

Barkley, R. A. (2013). *Taking charge of ADHD: The complete authoritative guide for parents* (3rd ed.). New York, NY: Guilford Press.

Parker, H. (2006). *The ADHD workbook for parents: A guide for parents of children ages 2–12 with ADHD*. Plantation, FL: Specialty Press.

Lesson 8

Babyak, M., Blumenthal, J. A., & Herman, S. (2000). Exercise treatment for major depression: Maintenance of therapeutic benefit at 10 months. *Psychosomatic Medicine, 62,* 633–638.

Blumenthal, J. A., Babyak, M. A., & Moore, K. A. (1999). Effects of exercise training on older people with major depression. *Archives of Internal Medicine, 159,* 2349–2356.

Bronson, P., & Merryman, A. (2009). *Nurture shock: New thinking about children.* New York, NY: Twelve.

Coopersmith, S. (1981). *The antecedents of self-esteem* (2nd ed.). Palo Alto, CA: Consulting Psychologist Press.

Jaycox, L., Reivich, K., Gillham, J., & Seligman, M. E. P. (1994). Prevention of depressive symptoms in school children. *Behavior Research & Therapy, 32,* 801–816.

Seligman, M. E. P. (2006). *Learned optimism: How to change your mind and your life.* New York, NY: Vintage Press.

Lesson 9

Faber, A., & Mazlish, E. (2012). *How to talk so kids will listen & listen so kids will talk.* New York, NY: Simon & Schuster.

Greene, R. W., & Ablon, J. S. (2006). *Treating explosive kids: The collaborative problem-solving approach.* New York, NY: Guilford Press.

Lesson 10

Baer, S., Saran, K., & Green, D. A. (2012). Computer/gaming use in youth: Correlations among use, addition, and functional impairment. *Paediatric and Child Health, 17,* 427–431.

Carr, N. (2010). *The shallows: What the Internet is doing to our brains.* New York, NY: Norton.

Gilbert, P. (2009). *The compassionate mind.* New York, NY: New Harbinger.

Monastra, V. J. (in press). *Teaching life skills to children and teens with ADHD.* Washington, DC: American Psychological Association.

Sax, L. (2007). *Boys adrift.* New York, NY: Basic Books.

Seligman, M. E. P. (2011). *Flourish: A visionary new understanding of happiness and well-being.* New York, NY: Free Press.

Lesson 11

Barkley, R. A. (2010). *Taking charge of adult ADHD.* New York, NY: Guilford Press.

Enright, R. D. (2012). *The forgiving life: A pathway to overcoming resentment and creating a legacy of love.* Washington, DC: American Psychological Association.

Hallowell, E. M., & Ratey, J. J. (2005). *Delivered from distraction: Getting the most out of life with attention deficit disorder.* New York, NY: Anchor Books.

Hallowell, E. M., & Ratey, J. J. (2011). *Driven to distraction: Recognizing and coping with attention deficit disorder* (rev. ed.). New York, NY: Anchor Books.

Levrini, A., & Prevatt, F. (2012). *Succeeding with adult ADHD: Daily strategies to help you achieve your goals and manage your life.* Washington, DC: American Psychological Association.

INDEX

ABOUT THE AUTHOR

Vincent J. Monastra, PhD, is a clinical psychologist and director of the FPI Attention Disorders Clinic in Endicott, New York. During the past 25 years, he has conducted a series of studies involving thousands of individuals with disorders of attention and behavioral control. He is the coinventor of the electroencephalograph (EEG)-based process approved by the U.S. Food and Drug Administration for use in the diagnosis of attention-deficit/hyperactivity disorder (ADHD), a pioneer in the development of parenting and EEG-based attention-training procedures, and the author of numerous scientific articles and book chapters. The first edition of his parenting book was named Parenting Book of the Year, and his book *Unlocking the Potential of Patients With ADHD: A Model for Clinical Practice* (2008), provides a model for comprehensive, effective, and practical community-based care for patients with ADHD. His skills as a master diagnostician and therapist have been internationally recognized and are archived in several educational videotaped programs, including *Working With Children With ADHD* (2005). He has been a faculty member of Wilson Hospital's Family Practice Residency Program, the Department of Psychology at Binghamton University, and most recently the Graduate School of Counseling and Clinical Psychology at Marywood University. He is the recipient of several scientific awards, including the President's Award and the Hans Berger Award for his seminal research into the neurophysiological characteristics of ADHD and his groundbreaking study on EEG biofeedback. He was listed among the country's most innovative researchers in the *Reader's Digest* 2004 edition of "Medical Breakthroughs." He can be contacted at www.drvincemonastra.com.